THE SIMPLY FIT DIET

Tim Covell

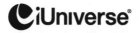

THE SIMPLY FIT DIET

iUniverse books may be ordered through booksellers or by contacting:

iUniverse
1663 Liberty Drive
Bloomington, IN 47403
www.iuniverse.com
1-800-Authors (1-800-288-4677)

ISBN: 978-1-4917-5034-6 (sc)
ISBN: 978-1-4917-5035-3 (e)

Printed in the United States of America.

iUniverse rev. date: 10/08/2014

THE SIMPLY FIT DIET

Tim Covell

The Simply Fit Diet™
All rights reserved © 2014

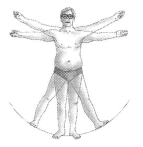

With special thanks to M. Lee, who created
the original artwork for this book.

Visit us online at TheSimplyFitDiet.com

Disclaimer:

This book is for healthy adults who are not and will not become pregnant. It is for information and discussion purposes only. **Nothing in this book is medical advice.** For medical advice, see a physician or other qualified health care professional. Always seek professional advice before starting a diet or exercise program.

Contents

Introduction

I am the fattest kid from a fat family. Like you, I have struggled with weight for my entire life. I have complained, aloud and to myself, how unfair it is that some people eat like pigs and stay thin, while I eat carefully and get fat. As a fat kid, my future health picture was grim. Fat children are all but destined to become fat adults and have a substantially increased risk of cardiovascular disease, diabetes, cancer, arthritis, sleep apnea, as well as social and psychological problems.

Facing this dilemma, my strategy was to eat relatively well and to be *very* active. I struggled to maintain my weight for years, but as I turned 50, my body was less able to tolerate the strain of constant exercise. At 50, I found myself with a sprained back, taking two prescription medications and three over-the-counter pills, with my weight creeping upward and my blood tests pointing toward a future of cardiovascular disease and diabetes. My doctor recommended statin drugs like Lipitor, but after researching the side effects, I decided not to take another pill.

About the same time, my brother went to the hospital to have his lower leg amputated as a result of diabetes. Until the amputation, his diabetes was undiagnosed. However, it should not have been a surprise. My father, who died at age 73, had diabetes. My oldest brother, 16 years my senior, has diabetes. Now, my second oldest brother, nine years my senior, lost his leg. That got my attention. In a few years, it would be me.

In the past, fitness was about looking good, with a general goal of being healthy. But facing the possibility of losing my mobility, or losing my life, fitness became my top priority.

Like you, I have read dozens of diet books and tried dozens of diets, all with limited success. I wondered if fitness could really be as difficult and unobtainable as it seemed. Despite eating well and exercising frequently, my future was bleak. I wondered if there was some simple solution that I was overlooking. There was.

Today, I have lost 40 pounds. I take no prescription medications and only an occasional aspirin or antihistamine. My blood work shows a lower than average risk of diabetes and cardiovascular disease. I take no nutritional supplements. I shop at regular grocers. I enjoy food more than I have in years. When I look at myself in the mirror, I hardly recognize myself. I have always struggled with being fat, hiding my body under baggy layers of full-cut clothes. Now I am slim. I wear the same size pants I wore at age 21. I sleep better and have as much energy as I did twenty years ago.

My path from being overweight and unhealthy to slim and healthy was not complex. It was simple. I am writing this to share the steps. By following the core concepts, you too can become simply fit.

The Simply Fit Diet is free. It is completely natural. It does not involve buying supplements, following complicated meal plans, or engaging in exhaustive exercise routines. You do not need to shop at specialty stores or consume foods you dislike. You do not need to count calories or measure portions. The food choices are diverse enough to suit the most confirmed carnivore as well as the most virtuous vegan. If you choose to follow the simple rules of this program, you will lose weight, feel better and become more healthy.

These seem like heady promises, and they are. You have been disappointed by numerous books and programs that promised similar results, but failed. I understand your skepticism. But think of it this way, following the standard dietary recommendations to lose weight is like trying to change a spark plug with a hammer. It is virtually impossible. The Simply Fit Diet, however, gives you the proper tools to accomplish your goals. With a ratchet and socket, changing a spark plug is easy. Similarly, with the right tools, becoming healthy will be surprisingly easy.

7

I will do my best in this book to provide you with techniques to change your perspective and achieve fitness. I will use a "shotgun" approach, making numerous suggestions and hoping they work for you. For example, as you begin your weight loss journey, I suggest that before every meal you grab a handful of your body fat, and say to yourself, "this is why I need to diet." If you find that too inconvenient, uncomfortable, or just plain silly, skip it. It is part of my shotgun approach to focusing your attention on health, but it is not essential to becoming fit. Just stick to the core concepts and you will accomplish your goal. Good luck on your journey.

The term "fat."

"Fat" is a stern term. It is usually used in a negative manner, for example, "he's so fat, how does he expect to get a date?" The official scientific terms are "overweight" and "obese," linked to specific body mass index calculations. Socially, terms like "husky," "large," "full-figured" and "big" are used to take some of the sting away from the label. But I use the term "fat" frequently in this book. It is clearly descriptive and it is honest. Further, many fat people want to deny that they are fat. If you do not admit you are fat, you will not face the truth and make the decision to become healthy. Hopefully, my using the direct term will make denial a little more difficult and help you to face reality.

The wild claims of diet books.

When you pick up a diet book, a preliminary question should be, was the author fat, and if so, did the program work for him? I am not anti-Atkins. However, Dr. Atkins built a moneymaking empire on his diet advice. When he died of questionable causes (allegedly due to a fall, but also perhaps from a stroke or heart attack) his empire had a significant financial interest in saying he was healthy–that his diet program worked. However, his death certificate lists his weight as 258 pounds; which, according to government guidelines for a six-foot tall

---

8

man, gave him a BMI of 35, well into the obese range. The Atkins diet may work in the short-run. It may work for some people in the long run, but for the founder and financial beneficiary of the Atkins empire, it did not keep him from dying an obese man. Similarly, health guru Dr. Andrew Weil makes millions on his books and health products. He does not reveal his weight or BMI, but his round belly and beard make him look like Santa Claus and photos of him in a hot tub leave little doubt that he is fat.

Some diet book authors, especially those who have come up in the fitness industry, are rumored to be steroid users. In my experience if you think someone might be using steroids, they are. The hypocrisy of achieving muscularity through drug use and then pretending others can achieve the same results without drugs is pervasive, from the local health club, to reality TV, and on the bestseller list. Steroid users are cheaters and their dishonest sales pitch should be ignored.

Other diet authors have never been fat. Vegans Neal Barnard and Joel Fuhrman give heartfelt nutrition counseling, but both appear to be naturally slim. Barnard was a college athlete and Furhman was a world champion figure skater. It is harder to trust their message when they do not really need it.

One of the biggest red flags in the diet industry is the products the author or program is selling. If they are selling supplements and meal plans, be careful. The endorsement of the Vegan Formula Mega Weight-Cutting Dietary Supplement may not be because it helps people lose weight, but because it makes the endorser more money.

Diet books make lots of wild claims, many of them on the cover. Here are a few:

- 4 Weeks, 20 pounds
- Lose up to 5 pounds in 5 days by eating the foods you love
- Kick start your metabolism and safely lose up to 10 pounds in 7 days

The wildest I have seen so far is the promise to lose eight pounds in three days. Now, losing a pound of weight means reducing your calorie intake by about 3,500. If you eat an average of 2,400 calories a day, *even if you ate nothing at all*, it would take more than eleven days to lose eight pounds. Books that promise unbelievable weight loss progress and use magic potions belong in the fiction section. Weight loss cannot be achieved with magic, it takes work.

Diet books are full of promises. I often joke that they not only promise glowing skin, elimination of all medications, cures for soreness and the effects of aging, but also that you will have to hire a lawyer to get an injunction to stop all the super-models who are pursuing you to get dates.

Some diet books are very convincing. When you read an Atkins diet book, it seems that meat is the only solution. But reading a vegan book convinces you of the opposite. The selectively cited science in each book supports the author's premise, but in fact science is not really sure what diets work and even less sure of why. If the answer were clear, the government would endorse and promote a diet plan and we would be a slim nation. But we are not. The truth of the matter is the scientists do not know why some diets work, and neither do I. I am not immune from the temptation to cite a little science in support of my diet, but I will try to limit it to science about what works, not explanations of why it works. I will also try to include some common sense, something we seem to have abandoned with disastrous consequences when we allowed scientists to tell us how to eat. Science started dominating the diet discussion in the 1960's and since that time the percentage of obese adults in the U.S. has increased from 13% to 36%. It is time to let common sense back into the discussion. In the old days, common sense led us to eat a salad or steak with black coffee as a diet meal. Science gave us low-fat TV dinners, diet soda and Snackwells that actually made us fatter. It is time for something different.

Here is the bottom line, The Simply Fit Diet works. The Simply Fit Diet is free. There are no Simply Fit Diet endorsed products and there never will be. The Simply Fit Diet is my honest explanation of a diet that worked for me and will work for you. Give it a try. You have nothing to lose but your excess weight and a world of health to gain.

Section One.
CHOOSE TO LOSE

Chapter 1. The Problem

If you have not looked at the most recent statistics about weight and health, you will likely find the results staggering. An unbelievable **74% of American men and 64% of women are overweight or obese, about 70% of the combined adult population**.

Currently, "body mass index"(BMI) is the popular shorthand for determining if someone is overweight (a BMI of 25 and over), obese (a BMI of 30 and over) or extremely obese (a BMI of 40 and over). For example, at 5'9" tall, my current weight of 148 produces a BMI of 21.85, in the healthy range. If I weighed between 169 and 202, I would be considered overweight. A weight of 203 would categorize me as obese, and a weight of 270 would make me extremely obese. For Americans, 36% of both men and women are obese, and the fastest growing group–literally–are the extremely obese. Currently, 8% of women and 4% of men are extremely obese.

Calculate your BMI.

You can find your BMI using the chart on page 48. Alternatively, you can calculate your BMI, either by using the formula (weight/(height in inches x height in inches)) x 703; or as a word problem, divide your weight by the sum of your height in inches times your height in inches. Multiply that total by 703 to find your BMI.

You can also go online to a site like http://www.cdc.gov/healthyweight/assessing/bmi/. BMI is a convenient guideline for categorizing large numbers of people without regard to their sex or build.

The concept of shape.

An alternative to the scientific calculation of BMI is the simple concept of shape. We use the term frequently, complaining that we are out of shape or need to get into shape. The concept has value. If you think of Leonardo da Vinci's 1490 diagram of man (Figure 1) as a healthy outline of the human shape, you can measure yourself against it to see how out of shape you have become. The average American man found on the bottom in Figure 1, is 5'9" tall, weighs 200 pounds and has a 40-inch waist. The average American woman is about 5'3" tall, weighs 166 pounds and has a 37.5-inch waist. The average American is not in shape.

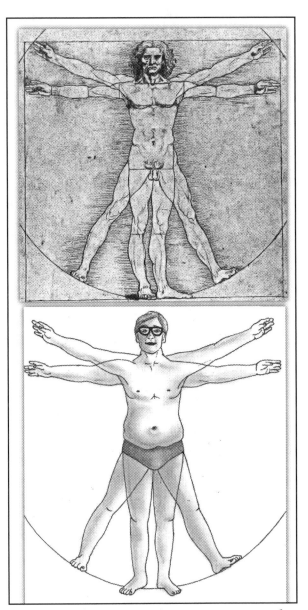

Figure 1. *The average American, compared to Da Vinci's 1490 drawing, is not in shape.*

The concept of shape also includes waist size, probably a more important indicator of health than BMI. The wider your waist, the higher your chance of disease. Note the difference in the waist of da Vinci's drawing and the average American man.

The concept of shape extends beyond our bodies and to our faces. We have so much excess fat that the terms apple or pear apply not only to our bodies, but to the shape of our obese faces as well. A mere 30 pounds separates the two photos of me in Figure 2, but the weight shows clearly in my face.

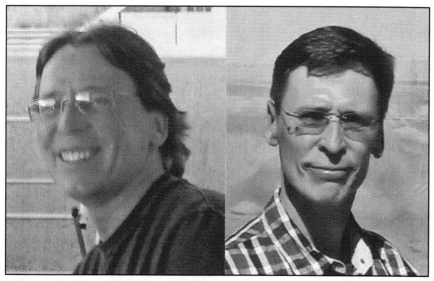

Figure 2. I am only 30 pounds heavier in the photo on the left, but the weight clearly shows in my face.

I am confident you have experienced meeting a person who is so far out of shape that it is uncomfortable to even look at him, that his body has gone so far beyond the bounds of an ordinary shape that it looks like he is about to burst. You do not need to calculate his BMI to know he is unhealthy. Scientific formulas like BMI can be clinical and hard to relate to. No math or formulas are needed for you to evaluate whether you are in shape.

A growing problem.

The expansion of Americans' waistlines in recent years has been remarkable. For example, at age 12 when my picture was taken in 1970 (Figure 3), just 4% of similar age children were obese. That is about one obese child in a class of 25. Currently, 33% of similar aged boys

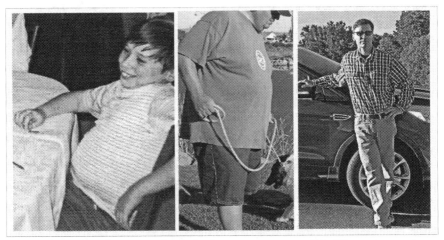

Figure 3. *The photo on the left shows me at age 12. The center photo is a sibling (and not the heaviest sibling) showing my genetic potential. The photo on the right is me today.*

are overweight and about 19% are obese, an almost five fold increase from when I was a child (for girls, the numbers are not much better, currently 30% are overweight and 15% are obese).

For American adults, the results are even more alarming. Obesity maps of the United States, which you can find animated online at http://www.cdc.gov/obesity/data/adult.html, show the trend graphically (Figure 4). In 1990, no state had an obesity rate *over* 15%.

1990

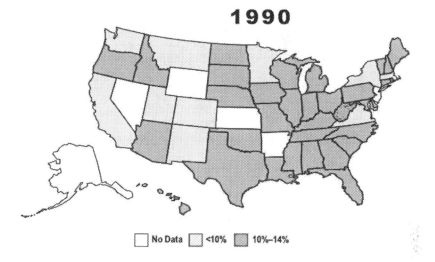

2012

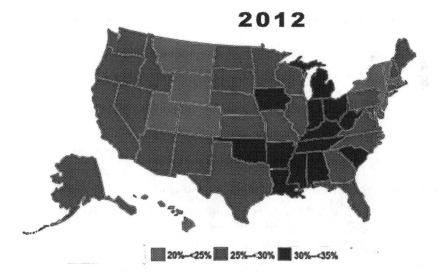

Figure 4. *Obesity in the United States is a growing problem.*

17

In 2012, no state had an obesity rate *under* 20%, nine states and the District of Colombia had a rate of 20-25% and thirteen states had a rate of 30% or more with Mississippi topping the chart at 34.6%.[1] Despite our societal focus on health, we keep getting fatter.

The problem with fat.

From a common sense perspective, being fat is not only unsightly, it is unhealthy. Think about all the extra work your body must do to maintain the excess pounds. Your body must provide your fat with nutrition and waste disposal. In addition, your bones and muscles must lug around the weight. Think of the stress 40 pounds in the belly puts on your back, knees and ankles. No wonder so many heavy people walk with difficulty. It is kind of like a city that has grown faster than its infrastructure. Surely you have been to a city where the population grew too fast and the highways are clogged with bumper-to-bumper traffic. Emergency vehicles like ambulances get caught in the traffic and fail to provide services in a timely manner. Electrical grids get overloaded and on high use days there may not be enough energy to go around. Science tells us that the same kinds of things happen to an overweight body.

Take diabetes for example. Diabetes is a term applied to two distinct diseases. Type 1 diabetes, sometimes called juvenile diabetes, is where the pancreas does not produce enough insulin. Only about 5% of diabetics have type 1 diabetes. The other 95% have type 2. Type 2 diabetes, sometimes called adult onset diabetes, is where the body, due to heredity and weight, stops responding to insulin, resulting in a host of problems.

Diabetes and the five miles per hour bumper.

I think of diabetes with this analogy. Imagine that as a young person you move to the city and rent an apartment in a high rise building. You park in the basement facing a concrete barrier. One evening, being young and foolish, you decide to try out your car's claim that you can crash at five miles per hour with no damage. You drive headlong into the concrete barrier to test the bumper. Sure enough, other than some flaked paint, there is no real damage. That is kind of like what you do to your body's insulin system after a late night of drinking beer, topped off with two hours of sleep and a breakfast of pancakes with syrup, washed down with a sweet coffee drink. Doing this once probably will not hurt your car and probably will not hurt your body. But imagine if you ram into the concrete barrier every time you come home. Eventually the car's shock absorbing system will fail, the car will begin to crumble, and you will crack your radiator or do some other damage that stops the car from running. Similarly, continually challenging your body with high doses of sugar and unhealthful foods results in a drop in insulin sensitivity, as shown by higher blood sugar test results, the primary diagnostic indication of pre-diabetes and diabetes.

The government provides a list of the top sources of calories in the diet of the average American youth. Excluding chicken, the top ten are:

- Grain-based desserts
- Pizza
- Soda/energy/sport drinks
- Yeast breads
- Pasta and pasta dishes
- Reduced-fat milk
- Dairy desserts
- Potato/corn/other chips
- Ready to eat cereals
- Tortillas, burritos and tacos

If you are an adult and your diet looks like that of an American youth, you are almost surely heading for a crash. Now, there is a saying that there is no one more holy than a reformed sinner, and that saying applies to me. For years, pizza was my favorite food, and on an almost daily basis I would have a soda plus a candy bar or cookie. Did I damage my body by eating poorly? Probably. Can the damage be reversed? I hope so.

Luckily, the car crash analogy is limited in its application to the human body. A car cannot repair itself, but the body, if not too badly damaged, can. Although in years past my annual health checkups indicated I was more likely than average to suffer from disease, since I adopted the Simply Fit Diet, my doctor tells me I am less likely than average to have diabetes and less likely than average to develop cardiovascular disease. When someone asks me if eating one donut will really hurt, I ask myself if I am willing to have my foot amputated from the complications of diabetes in trade for a donut. No donut or other sweet treat is worth the risk of losing my health.

Before I understood my risk for diabetes, I only knew generally that it was a bad disease that sometimes resulted in blindness and amputations. But increased knowledge has led me to see that the disease has even worse effects and also that for most it is preventable and treatable, not by medications, but by diet!

The explosion of diabetes among Americans is shocking, but goes hand in hand with the increase in obesity. Currently, **11.3% of the adult population has diabetes**, that is more than one in ten of the people you see on the street. A shocking **35% of the adult population has pre-diabetes**, a condition which if not addressed will lead to diabetes. Further, 50% of people over age 65 have pre-diabetes. Studies predict that within ten years, 77% of adult men and 53% of adult women will have diabetes or pre-diabetes.

Diabetes is an underlying contributor to a host of diseases. Diabetes can decrease life expectancy by as much as eight years and seriously decrease the quality of life.

The American Diabetes Association says that:

- Two out of three people with diabetes die of heart disease or stroke
- Diabetes is the leading cause of kidney failure
- Diabetes is the leading cause of new cases of blindness among adults
- The rate of amputation for people with diabetes is ten times higher than for people without diabetes
- About 70% of people with diabetes have mild to severe forms of nerve damage that could result in pain in the feet or hands, slowed digestion, sexual dysfunction and other nerve problems

The good news is that reducing your weight by as little as 7% (12 pounds for a 175-pound person) and increasing physical activity can significantly reduce your risk of getting diabetes.

For identical twins who develop type 2 diabetes after age 40, the disease almost always affects both twins. But twins Tim and Paul Daly are an exception to the rule. At age 44, Paul Daly was diagnosed with diabetes. At 5'10", Paul weighed 220 pounds. His twin Tim, who was pre-diabetic, weighed 200. Tim became part of a research study about preventing diabetes. He was in a lifestyle intervention group that encouraged diet and exercise. Tim was encouraged to lose 7% of his body weight and to exercise 150 minutes a week. It worked. Despite being pre-diabetic and genetically headed for diabetes, 14 years have passed and he still does not have the disease. In fact, the study showed that **diet and exercise are twice as effective as medication in preventing the onset of diabetes**. Physicians are quick to prescribe medicine, but diet and exercise, key components of the Simply Fit Diet, are a simple, free and natural way to help prevent diabetes. **Losing 7% of your body weight can reduce your chance of diabetes by 60%**.

Being fat increases your risk of diseases of the heart and circulatory system. It is easy to focus on the link between obesity and diabetes, but even more people are affected by circulatory diseases like heart attacks, stroke, and high blood pressure. I always knew that high blood pressure was undesirable, but I never really thought about why. But this concept helped me understand. If you make your fist into a wide circle and blow through it, the air passes easily. But if you clench your fist to make the space small, it takes a lot more effort to move the air through the space. This is like the contrast between normal and high blood pressure. When your blood pressure is high, it indicates that the veins and arteries are clogged with plaque and the heart has to work harder to send blood to the places that need it. In my simplistic mind, I think of plaque as fat in the veins and arteries.

Almost every American has plaque. Starting in the Korean War, doctors found that even young soldiers had streaks of plaque in their circulatory systems. More recently, autopsies of children who died accidentally have shown that the plaque now appears in our youth. This plaque is a precursor to the circulatory events that lead to heart attack and stroke–similar events where blood is either blocked from the heart or brain.

In the past, scientists told us that once you had plaque deposits in your system, nothing could be done to reduce them. However some physicians, like vegan doctor Neal Barnard, have published strong evidence that clogged veins and arteries can be improved, and that improvement was accomplished with diet, not drugs.

Excess weight is directly linked to a host of diseases that decrease both how well you live and how long you live. Excess weight increases your chances of getting:

- Type 2 diabetes (11.3% of the population has diabetes and 35% has pre-diabetes)
- Cardiovascular disease (37% of the population is diagnosed with cardiovascular disease, but the warning signs appear in almost every American)

- Hypertension (34% of the population has hypertension and another 36% has pre-hypertension)
- Cancer (41% of the population will be diagnosed with cancer in their lifetimes)
- Osteoporosis (50% of women and 25% of men will have an osteoporosis related fracture in their lifetimes)
- Stroke (5% of Americans will die of stroke)
- Dementia/Alzheimer's (33% of seniors die with dementia, 50% of people over 85 have dementia)
- Fatty liver disease (between 15% and 20% of Americans have some fatty liver disease, but 90% of obese people and 50% of diabetics have the disease)
- Sleep Apnea (About 4% of adult men and 2% of adult women are diagnosed with sleep apnea, and many more are undiagnosed)

You only get one body. If you damage your body with bad food and bad habits, it may well be too late to do anything about it. The time to act is now, not when you are struck by disease.

The democratization of medical information.

It used to be that you needed to go to a doctor to check your blood pressure or blood sugar. Nowadays, for modest cost, you can purchase machines to check these levels at home. A home blood pressure cuff costs less than $40, and a home blood sugar test machine costs around $15. These machines may not have the accuracy of a doctor's office or lab (blood sugar tests can be off by as much as 20 points) but they can give you an indication of how you are doing between doctor visits.

Years ago, Americans became aware of the risk of increased weight, and a whole new industry sprang up to help them control it. But after 50 years, the program appears to have failed.

It is not too difficult to figure out how we have gotten where we are–a fat nation. The other day I was in a fast food restaurant (eating a virtuous salad), when I saw an extremely obese woman eating chicken nuggets. She was a perfect example of how we have ended up where we are. Two hundred years ago, the fast and easy calories she was consuming were not available. Even if she wanted to have fried chicken 200 years ago, she would have had to chase down the chicken, pluck it and butcher it. She would have needed to gather wood and put a fire in the stove, and then to pan fry the chicken. Cleaning the cooking utensils and dishes would have been another chore, involving drawing water from a well and hand scrubbing the pots and pans. A fried chicken dinner 200 years ago would have involved a heck of a lot more physical effort and probably also produced a healthier meal.

Today, for only a few dollars, you can go to a fast food restaurant and get a disease inducing meal with minimal effort. You do not even need to get out of your car. Press the button on your power window and the food will be handed to you. No need to do the dishes, just drop the refuse in the special can with a neck extended so that drive-through customers do not even need to get out of their cars.

Heck, even in my youth there were fast food stands, but you had to walk to them to get your food. Most of the cars of my youth had manual transmissions, manual steering and crank windows. Now cars have power steering, one-touch up and down windows and the newest innovation, push button start where you do not even need to take a key from your pocket and twist the ignition, you just push a start button.

We even keep the temperature in our environment at a comfortable 70 degrees. Two hundred years ago, when there was no central air conditioning or heat, your body would burn extra calories staying warm on a cold day. Today, even that basic caloric expenditure is unnecessary.

We are living in a virtual horn of plenty, bordered on one side by cheap, easy, unhealthful calories galore, and on the other side by decreased physical activity (Figure 5). The result is a system that spits out overweight, unhealthy people who decrease their life expectancy and quality of life. It is not surprising that we have become fat.

A basic premise of this book is that fat on the outside is an indicator of fat on the inside. That fat surrounds and permeates the organs, it coats the insides of the veins and arteries and throws off the body's delicate chemical balance. Fat out means fat in. Fat causes or exacerbates a host of harmful diseases. Fat is bad. The solution is to lose weight, and that can be accomplished by eating healthy food and increasing your activity level. In its simplest form, we must narrow the horn of plenty (Figure 6).

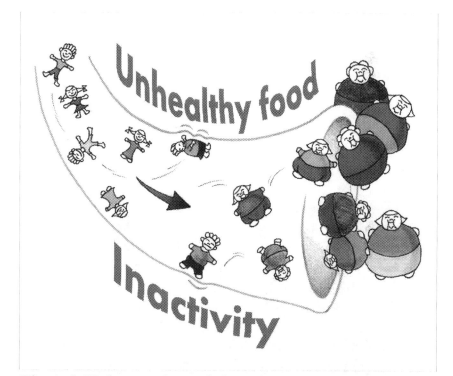

Figure 5. *We live in a horn of plenty, bouncing between unhealthy food and inactivity and emerging fat and sick.*

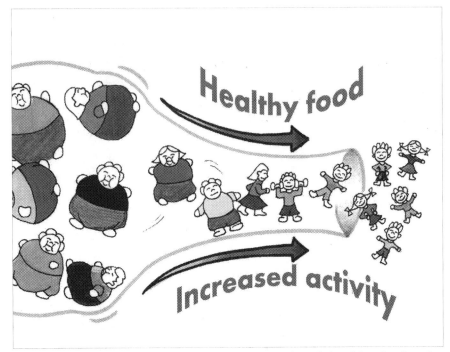

Figure 6. *The horn of plenty can be reversed with healthy food and increased activity.*

The goal of becoming fit is not to live longer, but to live better. Currently, two of my siblings cannot walk normally because of obesity related illnesses. One has lost his leg and another is so obese that unassisted walking is impossible. By following the Simply Fit Diet, I am able to walk, climb stairs, run, swim, bicycle, and most important, to enjoy my life. You can too.

The limits of vanity.
Vanity can be a strong motivating factor in weight loss, and I am happy to use it as a tool. However, with almost 70% of American adults overweight or obese, it is obvious that vanity is not enough. Making weight loss a matter of life or death provides a stronger

motivation for getting fit. As you lose weight on the Simply Fit Diet, you will likely use vanity as a motivating factor, but I encourage you to remind yourself that although looking good is a byproduct of this program, health is the most important long-term goal.

Chapter 2. Let's Talk About You

So far, I have talked about myself and the general American population. Now it is time to talk about you.

In preparation for the upcoming chapters, I am going to ask you to complete a few exercises. We will use them later in the book. Please really write down your answers, the process of thinking and committing the words to writing has more impact than just imagining your answers.

First, make a list of ten major life goals. Do not over-think them, just write down things that are on your mind at this point in your life. You may want to: dance at your daughter's wedding, ride the Trans-Siberian Railway, hike to the bottom of the Grand Canyon, earn a Master's degree, write a book, pay off your house, buy a Corvette, or whatever else is important to you.

Life Goals

1.	
2.	
3.	
4.	
5.	
6.	
7.	
8.	
9.	
10.	

Now, make a list of your ten favorite foods–even if they are bad for you. These are the foods that you would love to eat in a perfect world where you are trim and fit and food does not make you fat. I am not talking about a list that will make a nutritionist happy, but an honest list of the foods you love to eat when health and calories are not a concern.

My list looks like this:

1. Pizza
2. Beer and pretzels
3. Mashed potatoes with butter and sour cream
4. Macaroni and cheese
5. Lasagna
6. Chicken enchiladas
7. Chips or crackers and dip
8. Pancakes with butter and syrup
9. Donuts
10. Pasta with sauce

Don't forget the sauce.

Both in making your list of favorite foods and in deciding what foods to eat, do not forget that sauces, dressings and side dishes can be a significant component of the main dish. For example, at a popular chain restaurant a seven-ounce house sirloin has 280 calories. Make it a seven-ounce "Citrus Lime Sirloin," by adding some dressing, and the calories more than double to 570. Similarly, the amount of fat more than doubles, as does the sodium, and the carb count goes from one gram to 33.[2] At McDonald's, a Premium Bacon Ranch Salad has 140 calories, but add a packet of Ranch Dressing and the calorie count jumps to 310 while the fat content more than triples. Hot Cakes at the same restaurant sound pretty innocent at 350 calories, but add the obligatory syrup and two pats of margarine, and the dish jumps to 570

> calories. Sauces, dressings and sides can be a significant component of your meal.

Make your list of favorite foods here. Be sure to include the sauces and sides. For the time being, ignore the boxes that appear before your favorite foods.

My Favorite Foods

				1.
				2.
				3.
				4.
				5.
				6.
				7.
				8.
				9.
				10.

As a preliminary matter, look for patterns in your choice of favorite foods. Most people lean toward one type of food or another. For me, it is the combination of grains, oil and salt that makes pizza and lasagna so attractive. For others it is sugar combined with grain, or fried foods. Knowing these patterns will help you to identify your weaknesses. We will work with this list later in the book.

Next, think about the health issues of your siblings, parents and grandparents. Every family is different, yours might be subject to cancer, diabetes, stroke, heart attack, dementia, or a combination of diseases. Think of the people who are living with these diseases. Think of the people who have died. Then ask yourself, what are you doing to *not* suffer from disease the way that Mom, Grandpa, or Uncle Al did? What are you willing to do to *not* become that person? Look particularly closely at your parents. They represent your genetic destiny. **What are you doing to not become your parents?** We love to live in denial, but the reality is that without action, chances are you will suffer the same fate.

Now, go back to the list of life goals that you made earlier in this chapter. There is a space for a check mark next to each goal. Put a check next to every goal that you can accomplish *without* health.

Just about every goal requires health. Health cannot be taken for granted. However, this essential ingredient is often ignored. We put health on the back burner while we earn a living. We put health off to another day while we resolve relationship problems. We ignore health while we focus on family members. But we fail to realize health is essential to reach our goals. Health is essential to support our families. Investing in health cannot be put off while you work your way up the career ladder. You need health to climb that ladder. Health deserves as much time and attention as all those other issues you claim make you too busy to become healthy. You will not accomplish your goals or protect your family if you are dead. **Health is the most important thing in life.** All other goals follow from there.

Finally, in this chapter, I am going to tell you a couple of stories, and then ask yourself to imagine yourself in a particular situation. I am going to focus on diabetes, because it is an increasingly common disease and an underlying cause of many deaths. I am also focusing on it because it is dramatic and often results in a consequence short of death, one that I will ask you to imagine yourself facing.

Jazz singer Ella Fitzgerald was known as the first lady of song, winning 13 Grammy Awards, making more than 200 recordings, selling more than 40 million record albums and receiving honorary awards from two American Presidents. Always a large woman, Ms. Fitzgerald was diagnosed with type 2 diabetes in 1986. In 1991, she gave her farewell concert at New York's Carnegie Hall. In 1993, she had both legs amputated below the knee due to complications from diabetes. She never fully recovered from the amputation. Three years later, she died.

Born in Utah in 1944, Larry Miller was a car dealer and businessman whose business empire included car dealerships, radio and TV stations, movie theaters, the Utah Jazz basketball team, a minor league baseball team, and numerous companies and investments worth more than $480 million. Although athletic when young, Larry Miller was a big-bellied man. He was diagnosed with type 2 diabetes in the early 1990s. The diabetes caused a 2008 heart attack, kidney failure and in January 2009, he had both legs amputated six inches below the knee. Less than a month later, he died at age 64.

Both Ella Fitzgerald and Larry Miller were highly successful and wealthy. Both were overweight. Both developed a disease that could have been prevented by diet. On the day each faced amputation, what sum of money do you imagine they would have paid to keep their limbs? They certainly would have paid a million dollars, and most probably their entire net worth. Because it is a nice round sum, I am going to use the million-dollar figure. Would you pay a million dollars to keep your leg if you were facing amputation? I would. Conversely, if you can achieve fitness that allows you to keep your limb, you will effectively earn a million-dollars worth of health.

Now, think about the times you have been to the hospital. Think about the sights, smells and sounds. Were you at the hospital for treatment, or visiting a loved one? Think of why you or your loved one needed hospitalization. Other than child birth or accidents, for how many people did diet play a role in their being there?

Your hospital stay.

Imagine that years from now you have visited the doctor about problems with your right foot. Your diet has been far from perfect, but not all that bad, you tell yourself. You are overweight, but not grossly obese. But despite your rationalizations, your doctor tells you that things have gone too far and that you have a choice, to lose your life or lose your foot. The surgery must be conducted as soon as possible and you are admitted to the hospital overnight.

Close your eyes and count backward from 20 to one. As you count backward, relax, and release yourself to imagine this scene.

Imagine yourself reclining in a clean hospital bed. Listen to the beeping of the machines and the chatter of the nurses at the nurses' station down the hall. Think of the dull ache coming from your right foot and the incontrovertible evidence the doctor has presented that it must be removed to save your life.

Picture the things you use that foot for–driving, working, playing sports, climbing stairs. Think how difficult life will be, even with an artificial limb. Will you ever be able to run with your children or grandchildren? Will you be able to walk in the mountains and see the Fall colors? Will you be able to hop out of bed at night to check on a noise, or in a worse case scenario, to protect your family?

The leg must go, but ask yourself, if you could make a deal, what sum of money would you pay to keep it? If money could buy health, would you pay a million dollars to keep your leg? And more importantly, ask yourself what lifestyle changes would you make to keep that leg? Is there any food that you love so much, that you would lose your leg for it? Would you try any diet, even if sounded odd, if it allowed you to keep your leg? Think deeply about what losing a leg means to you.

Slowly count forward from one to 20, open your eyes and leave behind this exercise.

On the back cover of this book I made the wild claim that you could lose ten pounds in a day. The way to do it is not to diet, but to eat with abandon. Eat the foods on your favorites list without regard to the health consequences. Become obese. Ignore your doctor's warnings that you are becoming diabetic. Ignore your doctor's warnings about foot care. When your lower leg is amputated, you will lose about 6% of your weight, more than ten pounds for a 175-pound person. But I hope you will choose a better way to lose weight.

My father was a smoker for most of his life. Nothing made him quit. That is, until the day he received his cancer diagnosis. Without a word, he quit smoking and never smoked again. He always had the power to quit, he just never had the motivation.

Similarly, you have the power to become fit, you just have not made it your top priority. This book will provide you with the tools, but it cannot provide the motivation. Only you can do that. Asking yourself to imagine losing your leg–or losing your life–because of your health decisions introduces the first important premise of this book, that is to **make health a matter of life or death before it becomes a matter of life or death**.

The right time to become fit is right now. People are full of excuses about job stress, relationship stress and life stress. If you want a time without stress to improve your fitness, it may well never happen. The Simply Fit Diet takes no special effort. Some dietary changes are involved, but there is no counting calories, measuring portions or preparing difficult menus. You can eat all you want, and the food choices are easy. I will not even ask you to quit drinking alcohol or coffee! The most important decision you will make is the decision to become fit. Do not put it off. Start now.

Fat, fate and free will.

The concept of free will underpins our society. Therefore, it is natural to assume that people know they can choose to lose weight. However, a disturbing number of people (including some of my siblings) act as if fat is their fate. If you believe fat is your fate, you are unlikely to change. Perhaps accepting fat as your fate relieves you of the unpleasant recognition that you are fat because of the choices you have made. However, there are numerous examples of people who have lost weight, from me (see Figure 3), to reality show contestants, and probably the best example of all, the 10,000 people in the National Weight Control Registry who have lost an average of 66 pounds and kept it off for an average of 5.5 years.[3]

As you start your weight loss journey, I encourage you to consider whether you believe that fat is your fate, or whether you believe you can choose to lose. If you do not believe that you can achieve a healthy weight, it is unlikely that you will. By having your values and goals in alignment, you have the best chance of becoming fit. In order to choose to lose you must first believe you have a choice.

Section Two.
BUILD A FOUNDATION

Chapter 3. Setting the Stage

Face reality.

The explosion of obesity in the U.S. shown by the maps on page 17 is sobering. The maps graphically reflect America's growing obesity problem. But the maps *understate* the problem. The maps are based on self-reports. The surveyors telephone homes around the country and ask the height and weight of the people who answer. If someone surveyed you, would you tend to give an answer that reflected best upon you? Would you choose your lowest weight within the past month, and maybe strive to be a half-inch taller than you really are? Studies show that people tend to do both, they understate their weight and overstate their height.

Similarly, although almost 70% of adult Americans are either overweight or obese, a Gallup survey shows that 60% are perfectly satisfied with their weight. They do not believe that they should diet.

The same sort of denial exists on an individual level. Most fat people suffer from denial. Most do not step on the scale on a daily basis. They do not stand naked and look at themselves in the mirror. They avoid photographs that memorialize their health status. This reality avoidance makes it easier to continue doing what they are doing–and what they are doing is engaging in behavior that threatens their health.

If you are afraid to step on the scale or look in the mirror, you are denying reality. The first step toward improving your health is to honestly evaluate where you are now. The good news is that when you use the tools in this book, you will lose weight quickly. The record you make now will be a reference point to measure your improvement. The biggest step you have made is deciding to become healthy. A difficult step will be evaluating where you are now, but soon being overweight will be a thing of the past.

Take a good look at yourself.

As you lay the foundation for the Simply Fit Diet, you should stand naked in front of the mirror and take a good look at yourself. Do not imagine yourself doing this, actually do it. Bring along a hand mirror so that you can see the rear view as well. View yourself from the side. Do you look like a wood plank (a healthy state) or a barrel (a sign of obesity)? Does your stomach stick out more than your chest? Are there creases and folds on your belly? Do you have saddle bags on your sides? Has fat climbed up your chest and spread to your back, neck and face? All of these things will improve as you follow the Simply Fit Diet, but an honest self-evaluation will reinforce your resolve to change. For some people, a photograph is a more effective reflection of reality. Modern electronics make it easy to snap a photo of yourself and then to study it privately. **Taking a good look at yourself is an important way to start the Simply Fit Diet.**

The contours of fat.

When most people think of fat, they think of the rolls you see around the middle of so many Americans. Although these rolls are one of the most visible forms of fat, fat also accumulates within your rib cage, in your liver and internal organs and in other parts of the body.

The fat the scientists tell us is most dangerous is the fat that grows inside of your rib cage and drapes over the internal organs like an umbrella. You have probably seen someone with very little external fat, but with a bulging belly, as if the person swallowed a barrel. Such a person is a walking example of internal fat.

Even without knowing the dangerous health consequences of being fat, common sense shows that it is not healthy. Let's revisit the city analogy for a moment and imagine that your body is like a city. Your arteries provide nutrients to your body parts just the way the utilities provide power and water to homes in the city. Your body carries away waste just as the sewer system and garbage trucks do in a city. A well-planned city can provide all of the necessary services smoothly.

But imagine that you suddenly increase the population of the city by 37%. Suddenly the roads will clog with traffic. The emergency vehicles will have a hard time getting through. On stressfully hot or cold days, the utility services may become overloaded and you can suffer brownouts or reduced natural gas pressure.

The 37% population growth in a city is in many ways like the 55 pounds it would take for me to go from a healthy weight to obese. Those extra 55 pounds require nutrients and waste disposal just like the other cells of my body. My body will have to work harder to supply blood and oxygen to the new cells, and the liver and kidneys will need to deal with the increased waste.

Also, thinking logically, the extra 55 pounds will put significant stress on my ankles, legs and back. It is likely that I will have a harder time getting in and out of bed, and that I will feel sore and less likely to exercise.

But, your fat does not care about your sore ankles. Your fat does not care about your sore back. Your fat does not care that it makes it harder for you to exercise. Your fat does not care that it is streaking your arteries with plaque and that it is putting you on the course to diabetes, cardiovascular disease and other problems. **Your fat is in many ways a monster.**

Meet Audrey.

In the movie *Little Shop of Horrors*, a blood sucking plant named Audrey (Audrey II, to be precise, but for simplicity I will call her Audrey) caused havoc in the life of a plant store clerk named Seymour. In the dark comedy, the plant grew larger and larger demanding more and more blood and crying out, "feed me, Seymour!" It is not unreasonable to think of your fat as Audrey.

In fact, your relationship with Audrey is one sided and dysfunctional. Audrey does not care about you. She does not care about your health. She does not care about your sore back and sore ankles. She only cares about herself. Audrey wants you to feed her–an extra 1,025 calories a day for a man my size to support 55 excess pounds. Further, Audrey is not satisfied with what you feed her, she wants to grow!

Getting rid of Audrey is not as simple as showing her the door. She will hang around for months and she will not go quietly. She will beg and plead and scream, "feed me, Seymour." And in the case of the majority of Americans, she wins. She insists on being a part of you, even if your involvement with her will both shorten your life span and lower your quality of life (Figure 7).

Like in most dysfunctional relationships, Audrey makes

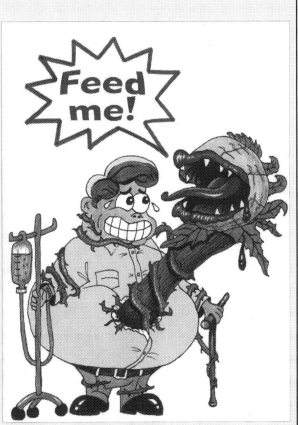

Figure 7. Your fat is like a foreign invader, seeking to grow, even though it hurts your health.

demands. So much of what you think of as hunger is really Audrey demanding to be fed. But her cravings and hunger are easily distinguished. If you are craving something from your list of favorite foods, it is almost certainly Audrey demanding to be fed. If you are hungry, your body will be satisfied by food, most any food, but particularly healthful, natural foods. An apple will do. Audrey, however, demands high-calorie, high-fat, high-carbohydrate treats. Do not let Audrey fool you that only fattening foods will work.

It may sound far fetched to describe fat as an evil intentioned foreign invader, but scientists are discovering information that makes this story more realistic. Scientists have discovered that fat secretes and alters body hormones. One of its purposes is to support and increase its size. Further, scientists have found that fat not only can change how your body functions, but can also change your brain. Those brain changes make you more likely to eat foods that, guess what, increase your body fat. The brain changes may be caused by inflammatory cells traveling to the hypothalamus. The brain is then unable to accurately sense the amount of fat being stored. A high-fat, high-carbohydrate diet causes your brain to think your fat stores are permanently empty, when in fact they are full. The good news is that the damage to the brain can be reversed by switching to a healthier diet

Audrey is very much like a foreign invader because her goal is her gain to your detriment. She has commandeered your body systems for her own purposes. She has sunk her roots into your chest, arms, face, heart and liver. To protect your health, you must evict her, but it won't be easy. The medicine you will have to take is healthy food, exercise, and yes, occasional hunger. But the cure is worth it.

Step on the scale.

Imagine driving down the highway in a speed enforcement zone. There are speed cameras and police officers giving out tickets. You are late for a meeting and you neither want to spend the time nor the money on a ticket. Would you look at your speedometer? Of course you would.

The consequences of being fat are more far reaching than getting a speeding ticket, but a huge number of people never look at the speedometer–in this case the scale–to monitor how they are doing.

Diet books and websites are full of recommendations about how *infrequently* you should weigh yourself. Some say weekly, others say monthly and a few say never. Why the myth that not weighing yourself is healthy began and why it is perpetuated is beyond me. What you weigh today is a reality you must face. What you weigh tomorrow is part of that reality. How your food and beverage consumption affects your weight is important. Of course your weight will vary from day to day. You should become familiar with the variance and face reality. What effect does drinking a liter of water have on your weight? Might as well find out. What happens to your weight when you go overboard and drink a six pack of beer and eat half a pizza? You did it, so face reality. If pigging out on pizza and beer causes you to gain three pounds, you might as well know it immediately, instead of waiting a week or month to see the results, and in which time you might repeat the experience three more times because you did not face the consequences the first time.

A number of studies show that people who weigh themselves daily take off weight more quickly and keep the weight off better. Daily weighing is a no-cost, low-effort way to maximize your weight loss. Just as the price of liberty is constant vigilance, the price of fitness is constant monitoring. A key aspect of the Simply Fit Diet, both when you are losing weight and later when you transition to maintaining your weight, is monitoring. **Recording your weight at least daily is a strategy you should adopt now and maintain for the rest of your life.**

Some common sense tips about weighing yourself.

To weigh yourself, you should have a good scale. Take your current scale and step on it three times. If the weights are the same or very close, great. Unfortunately, many old scales show results that vary by pounds. If your scale is inconsistent, buy a new one. Many modern electronic scales cost less than $40 and produce amazingly consistent results. Heck, if health is worth a million dollars then $40 is a small investment.

A further tip about the scale, be sure to put it in the same spot on a flat, hard floor. Bathroom floors often have squares and patterns. Choose a convenient spot, and then use the scale in the same spot every time. You can even mark the floor with some tape if you move the scale after every use. Similarly, put your feet on the same spot on the surface of the scale every time you weigh yourself and you will get more consistent results.

Always weigh yourself at the same time of day and wearing the same thing. Weighing yourself first thing in the morning when you are naked and ready to shower is a great time. To achieve greater consistency, use the restroom before you weigh yourself.

If you weigh yourself more than once a day, choose a weight to be your official weight. The first weight of the morning is usually the best. That is the weight you will tell your spouse and friends—and any surveyors who call for nationwide statistics.

If you weigh yourself more than once on each occasion, or if your scale jumps around a bit, choose a convention to select a consistent

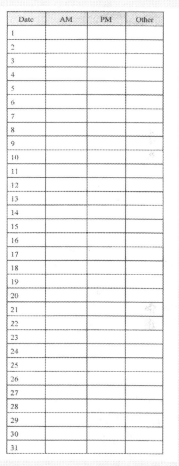

Figure 8. *A sample weight chart.*

weight. For example, always use the highest weight, or the lowest weight, or the middle weight of three tries.

Finally, record your weight. Keep a pen and paper, perhaps in a waterproof ziplock bag, near the scale. Figure 8 shows a sample weight chart that you can download from TheSimplyFitDiet.com. It is amazing how faulty memory is. With a written record, you can see what you weighed three months ago. You can see if your weight loss is slower or faster this month. And you can see if your bad choices are making you gain weight.

Weighing yourself daily will also be essential on the far end of your weight loss program. To lose weight, you will alter the content and quantity of food you eat. When you reach your weight goal, you will be able to add more food, or a wider variety of food, to your diet. Constant monitoring will allow you to quickly see the results of your experiments and to learn which foods you can add without gaining weight.

A final benefit of weighing yourself at least daily is that studies show people who weigh themselves regularly are more successful at losing weight and maintaining weight loss than those who do not. Whether the weigh-in acts as a goal setting exercise, or whether the constant monitoring limits binges, is not clear; but it works.

People watch.

Looking at other people can help you to lose weight. To do this exercise, find a day on which you have some spare time. Go to a public building visited by a cross-section of the population, somewhere like a mall, movie theater, or popular store. Find a bench out front, and watch the people walk in. How many of them look trim, fit and healthy? How many look fat and sick?

Pay particular attention to people your age. At almost any age you will observe people for whom obesity has become a burden. For older people, some resort to canes, walkers and wheelchairs. Pay particular attention to those in wheelchairs. For how many do you guess that obesity contributed directly or indirectly to their being in a wheelchair? Also observe how surprisingly young some people are whose fat makes walking difficult. Ask yourself, which kind of person do I want to be, the one who has a hard time walking, or the one who strides with energy and pride?

As I mentioned before, out of six children in my family, two have severe mobility limitations caused by obesity. Of the remaining siblings, all have some mobility limitations related to obesity. I do not seek to be fit to live longer, I just want to live better. I have made the choice to be healthy, and if you see me walking into the building, I will be striding with pride. After you observe the high rate of obesity and its harmful effects, you will be more likely to choose to be fit.

Match the food with the shopper.

A variation on the people watching exercise you can engage in every time you go to the grocery store is to match the contents of the shopping carts to the shoppers. Almost always you will find that the contents of the shopping cart explain the shape of the shopper. Fat people tend to have carts with soda, chips and convenience foods, while slim people tend to have carts with whole foods. This observation reinforces the fact that what you eat affects your health.

Set realistic written goals.

Imagine that for some reason you need to drive to the geographic center of America: Lebanon, Kansas. Without a map or a plan, you hop into your car and drive the speed limit all day. You can drive like crazy, but unless you know the roads to get there, you could be going in the wrong direction and at the end of the day, be further from your goal than when you started. Having clear, realistic goals draws you toward your destination in almost a magical manner. I suggest that you set weight loss goals and mile markers along the way.

Looking to TV and movies for role models leads to a terribly distorted view of how Americans should look. To start with, celebrities are selected because they are unusually good looking. Even the villains look good. Further, the people you see on TV are as much the products of drugs and plastic surgery as they are products of nature. It is unnatural for 50- and 60-year-old celebrities to be free of wrinkles and blemishes, but turn on the TV and you see them every night. It is unnatural for men on TV to have washboard abdomens and for women to have perfectly shaped lips, breasts and buttocks, but you see them every night.

Steer clear of steroids.

For men, but also for women, special mention must be made of the role of steroids in modern life. Anabolic steroids first appeared in Olympic-level sports in the late 1950's. Today, they have spread to even high school sports. An incredible 11% of high school boys and 7% of high school girls have tried steroids. Fifty percent of high school and college athletes take some kind of sports supplement. Sports stars like Lance Armstrong and Alex Rodriguez have joined actors like Arnold Schwartzenager and Sylvester Stalone in acknowledging, or being forced to acknowledge, that they have used steroids to gain an unfair advantage. Instead of labeling these people heroes or role models, we should call them what they are–cheaters.

Steroids permeate the fitness industry. Many of the media stars who promote fitness are cheaters. Many of the trainers at the local gym, both male and female, are cheaters. It is impossible to attain the degree of muscularity these cheaters maintain, without using the same methods. Steroid users are not admirable, they are pitiful. They jab needles into their rear ends and inject drugs upsetting the natural balance of their bodies and shutting down their normal hormone production. The reasons these people do this are likely complex and may be rooted in fragile self images and rough pasts. But the bottom line is that they are not admirable but pitiful. You should be careful to not let your image of health be distorted by steroid users at the gym or in the media.

I turned on the TV the other day and saw a promotional advertisement for a reality show in which a lineup of handsome young men competed for a marriage proposal from an attractive young woman. The ad featured all of these men shirtless and tanned. I was appalled to conclude that not one or two, but every single one of them used steroids. To find a more realistic picture of what men should look like, we can go back to the era before steroids were widely available. No one will question the masculinity of the soldiers who fought for America in World War II, but when you look at photos from that era, you will find the soldiers shockingly slim (Figure 9). Conversely, if you look at pin-up models from that era, you will likely conclude that women like Marilyn Monroe would be kicked off today's reality shows for being too fat. Our current culture is distorted by the use of drugs and plastic surgery. If you must look to celebrities for role models, you should ignore cheaters like Arnold Schwartzenager and Sylvester Stalone, and look instead at men built like Mick Jagger or Woody Allen. Natural is better. The current focus on muscularity is neither natural nor healthy.

Beauty bought with a needle or a knife is illusory. If your goal is to look like a movie star, you are consigned to failure. You have neither the genetics, nor the professional chef, performance enhancing

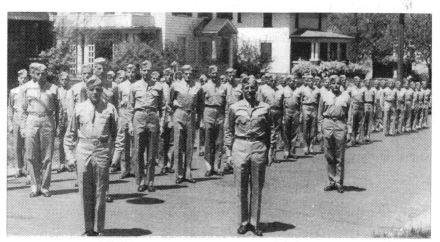

Figure 9. In the era before steroids, our heros were slim.

drugs and plastic surgery the movie star has. You need to set a realistic goal based on you, not based on someone you see in the movies or on TV.

Do not look to others for your weight goals, look to yourself. There was likely a time in your life when you were fit. This could have been in your late teens or twenties. Choose a time when your skeletal frame had grown to full size and remember your weight. *Even if decades have passed, that weight is still attainable.* Write down the most healthy weight you have been in your adult life. That will likely be your weight loss goal.

Some people have never been at a healthy weight. If this describes you, you can usually think of a relative of the same sex and a similar build who is or has been a healthy weight. Using someone with a similar genetic background can help you to target a healthy weight.

If you have never been a healthy weight and you have no relatives who are or have been at a healthy weight, you can use a BMI chart to set a goal (Figure 10). A BMI of 22 is generally considered a healthy weight. Or alternatively, seek out an old insurance height/weight chart[4] and use the weight suggested.

Beyond calculating these weights mentally, it is essential to write them down. When you write something down you process the numbers through a different part of your brain. You also make a written commitment to work toward your goals.

Height	BMI	21	22	23	24	25	26	27	28	29	30	31	32	33	34	35	36	37	38	39	40
5'0"		107	112	118	123	128	133	138	143	148	153	158	163	168	174	179	184	189	194	199	204
5'1"		111	116	122	127	132	137	143	148	153	158	164	169	174	180	185	190	195	201	206	211
5'2"		115	120	126	131	136	142	147	153	158	164	169	175	180	186	191	196	202	207	213	218
5'3"		118	124	130	135	141	146	152	158	163	169	175	180	186	191	197	203	208	214	220	225
5'4"		122	128	134	140	145	151	157	163	169	174	180	186	192	197	204	209	215	221	227	232
5'5"		126	132	138	144	150	156	162	168	174	180	186	192	198	204	210	216	222	228	234	240
5'6"		130	136	142	148	155	161	167	173	179	186	192	198	204	210	216	223	229	235	241	247
5'7"		134	140	146	153	159	166	172	178	185	191	198	204	211	217	223	230	236	242	249	255
5'8"		138	144	151	158	164	171	177	184	190	197	203	210	216	223	230	236	243	249	256	262
5'9"		142	149	155	162	169	176	182	189	196	203	209	216	223	230	236	243	250	257	263	270
5'10"		146	153	160	167	174	181	188	195	202	209	216	222	229	236	243	250	257	264	271	278
5'11"		150	157	165	172	179	186	193	200	208	215	222	229	236	243	250	257	265	272	279	286
60'''		154	162	169	177	184	191	199	206	213	221	228	235	242	250	258	265	272	279	287	294
6'1"		159	166	174	182	189	197	204	212	219	227	235	242	250	257	265	272	280	288	295	302
6'2"		163	171	179	186	194	202	210	218	225	233	241	249	256	264	272	280	287	295	303	311
6'3"		168	176	184	192	200	208	216	224	232	240	248	256	264	272	279	287	295	303	311	319

Figure 10. Body Mass Index chart.

How low can you go?

A recent study shows that medical costs begin rising progressively from a BMI of 19. For me to have a BMI of 19, I would weigh 128 pounds! Some people go even further. Focusing on science that shows rodents served a starvation diet live longer, calorie restriction (CR) proponents choose a similar course for themselves. It's a free country and people can choose the goals that make the most sense to them. With almost 70% of Americans being overweight or obese, I think a goal of maintaining a BMI of about 22, or alternatively, being in a shape similar to Leonardo da Vinci's picture of man (page 14), is enough.

Take a few minutes now to do some goal setting.

_____ Current weight.

_____ 93% of current weight (point at which the chance of diabetes is substantially reduced).

_____ Weight at BMI of 30 (dividing line between obese and overweight).

_____ Weight at BMI of 25 (dividing line between overweight and normal).

_____ Weight at BMI of 22.

_____ **Personal Weight Goal.**

$_____ One million dollars divided by (current weight minus goal weight) = how much value in health you earn with each pound lost.

_____ After you reach your weight goal, the highest weight you will accept before going back on the full Simply Fit Diet.

When I started my diet, my figures looked like this:

____190____ Current weight.

____177____ 93% of current weight (point at which the chance of diabetes is substantially reduced).

____203____ Weight at BMI of 30 (dividing line of obese and overweight).

____169____ Weight at BMI of 25 (dividing line of overweight and normal).

____149____ Weight at BMI of 22.

____**150**____ **Personal Weight Goal.**

$__25,000__ one million dollars divided by (current weight minus goal weight) = how much value in health you earn with each pound lost.

____160____ After you reach your weight goal, the highest weight you will accept before going back on the full Simply Fit Diet.

Being overweight is the result of a long series of bad choices. However, you have the power to reverse the bad choices by making better food and fitness choices. The body is naturally driven to heal. If you give it the right food and environment, it will do so. But it is slow. Weight loss is like steering an ocean liner–it takes time. It is easy to blame your weight gain on genetics, stress, work or family. But that is not going to make matters better. You must take responsibility for where you are now and the decisions you have made. It is easy to say that you will start a diet tomorrow, or on New Year's Day. But there are a limited number of tomorrows. One of these days they will be sawing your leg off and it will be too late. It is your decision to become fit and the time to act is right now.

Make a trip to the butcher.

Once you have calculated how much weight you would like to lose, stop by the butcher section of your grocery store. Assuming you have a bit of weight to lose, big box stores like Costco or Sam's Club work well for this exercise. Find the area with big packages of boneless meat. I like the approximately ten-pound tubes of pork they have at Costco. They look like an arm or leg. Gather together packages representing the amount of weight you want to lose and if possible, pick them up. Feel the mass and heft of the meat. Think of how much work it is to carry that weight everywhere you go. Think of how you look with that quantity of meat glued to your belly, hips and rear.

This exercise sounds a bit silly and would be very easy to skip, but it is extraordinarily beneficial. It makes concrete an abstract concept like losing 40 pounds. It helps you to both realize the burden the extra weight places on your body and the benefit of being free of it. It is also an exercise

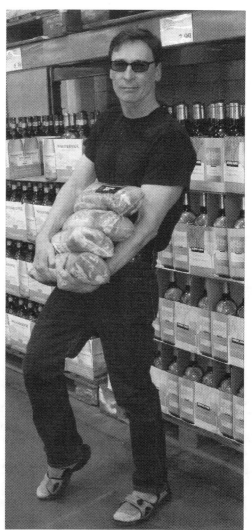

Figure 11. Struggling to lift packages of meat equal to the weight I lost encourages me to remain fit.

you should revisit after you lose some weight. After you have lost ten pounds, pick up a ten-pound piece of meat and feel its mass and heft (Figure 11). Feel proud that you no longer carry around this piece of meat. Think about the energy your body will save no longer needing to provide nutrients and waste disposal to the extra tissue. Most importantly of all, when you consider breaking your diet, ask yourself if what you think you will gain by eating unhealthy foods is worth plastering that ten-pound package of meat back on your body. **Holding the amount of weight you need to lose (or the weight you have already lost) and making it concrete will help you to reach your weight loss goals.**

Grab a handful of body fat before every meal.

This recommendation sounds strange, but it is highly effective. As you start your diet, before every meal, go to a private place, lift up your shirt and take a look at your fat. Say to yourself, "this is why I need to diet." You will **reinforce your goal of weight loss in a concrete way at least three times a day**. Alternatively, if you are not in a setting where you can do this, grab a handful of body fat before the meal and say the same thing. It is easy to get off track on a diet, especially at work or in social settings. Reminding yourself of your weight loss goal before every meal makes it easier to stay on track.

Get a good night's sleep.

It may sound strange to talk about sleep in a diet book, but sleeping well is essential for weight loss and health. If you think about it logically, sleep must be important to our bodies, we devote almost a third of our lives to it.

Scientists have long understood the relationship between healthy sleep and healthy weight. They tell us that a good night's sleep ensures essential hormones are secreted that affect not only what foods we desire during the daytime, but also how we metabolize them. Similarly, a poor night's sleep leads to cravings for high-sugar, high-carb foods, and encourages our bodies to turn meals into fat.

One of the most interesting studies I read was conducted in Boston where healthy volunteers were fed controlled meals and put in a sleep lab without clocks or windows, where the subjects' sleep cycles could be manipulated.[5] The subjects included both younger and older adults who lived in the sleep lab for five weeks. Diet, room temperature and exercise opportunities were all controlled. After sleeping on a normal schedule for six days, the subjects were put on a 28-hour day, with the opportunity for 6.53 hours of sleep, over a three-week period.

During sleep manipulation, the subjects experienced a 32% reduction in insulin secretion after meals, leading to inadequate glucose regulation. Some of the otherwise healthy subjects were becoming pre-diabetic. The sleep reduction also led to a reduction in metabolism, such that with no other changes, *a person would gain about 12.5 pounds a year simply by not sleeping well!* There was little difference in the negative effect of sleep deprivation based on the age of the subjects.

This highly controlled experiment using healthy subjects shows the importance of sleep in maintaining health and demonstrates that sleep deprivation can lead to diabetes and weight gain. The good news from the study is that with a nine-day sleep readjustment period, the harmful effects reversed. Applying these results to real life, **with as little as nine days of sleeping well, you can improve your health and lose weight with no other changes in lifestyle**.

A deep and restful sleep seems to come easily to young people, but is more and more difficult to obtain as one ages. I like to joke that the challenge of youth is to get a date, but the challenge of middle age is to get a good night's sleep.

The best way for you to improve your sleep is to make a good night's sleep a goal and to think logically about your individual situation and how to improve it. Preliminarily, you should set aside an adequate block of time to sleep. People like to boast about how little time they have to sleep, and for some it seems difficult to find more time. However, anyone who watches television or spends time on the internet or social media has little justification to say they cannot find time for sleep. Time is available, it is just not a priority. If you make sleep a more important priority, if you acknowledge sleep is essential to your health, you will allot an adequate amount of time for it.

For some, there is an adequate time for sleep, it is just difficult to fall asleep or stay asleep. Sometimes an active mind can keep you up at night. You may be worrying about a problem at work or a conflict with a family member. Keeping a journal at your bedside and writing about your concerns can sometimes give you adequate peace to fall asleep. Simple techniques like consciously relaxing can help. I like to count backwards from twenty to one, while imagining I am walking down a flight of stairs and with each step I become progressively more relaxed and sleepy. It is surprisingly effective.

Sometimes environmental factors hurt sleep. There may be light coming in through a window or from electronics in your room. Once again, common sense dictates a solution; perhaps a room darkening shade, or turning off or putting a box over a bright electronic device.

Pets can demand attention late at night, or their shifting and turning on the bed can wake you. Sometimes, despite your love for your pet, it is better to give your pet its own bed close to you, rather than have it rob you of sleep by sharing your bed.

Snoring is another problem, either yours or your spouse's. Snoring, unfortunately, is an indicator of sleep apnea, a much under-recognized condition that affects many overweight adults. Sleep apnea is where you stop breathing during your sleep. It can be caused either by a physical blockage in the throat, or an electronic problem in the body. When you stop breathing, your body awakens you with a start, reinitiating the breathing process but perhaps waking you a hundred times during the night and preventing you from getting the most deep, restful and healthful sleep. Sleep apnea is highly related to obesity. Even losing a small amount of weight can improve it significantly. Further, as discussed in Chapter 5, avoiding grains seems to improve the quality of sleep and may reduce the incidence of sleep apnea. By following the Simply Fit Diet you will significantly improve the quality of your sleep.

Alcohol consumption also hurts sleep. First, over-consumption of alcohol makes sleep apnea worse. Second, over-consumption of alcohol, even without sleep apnea, can make you sleepy in the short term, but the body puts alcohol first in line for processing and around four hours after going to bed you may awake from the heat and energy of the alcohol burning off. After that four-hour period alcohol acts as a stimulant that can make sleep difficult. You can reduce these negative effects by cutting your alcohol consumption or at least starting it earlier in the evening.

Caffeine consumption can also negatively affect sleep. The extra cup of coffee or other caffeinated beverage you consume for energy during the day can come back to haunt you with sleeplessness at night.

This often starts a negative cycle where you have even more caffeine the next day and sleep even more poorly the next night. Monitoring and reducing caffeine consumption, and limiting it to earlier hours, can help to improve sleep.

Liquid consumption, including coffee, tea, alcohol and other beverages can also interrupt your sleep cycle if you need to wake up to use the restroom. Consuming beverages earlier in the day and emptying your bladder fully right before bed can help. If you do need to use the restroom at night, use a gentle, indirect light, so as to make falling back asleep easier. Also, interestingly, many people with sleep apnea report they thought they rose at night to use the restroom when in fact they were being awakened by sleep apnea and then deciding to use the restroom since they were awake. Losing weight and improving your sleep apnea may well remedy a perceived need to use the restroom at night.

Napping can be a useful tool in getting enough rest. The body naturally lags after lunch. Most cultures in the world take a siesta. Only the industrialized North sought greater worker productivity by skipping this nap and many of us have learned to use caffeine and sugar to get through the early afternoon doldrums. Instead of resisting, if you have time, consider taking a nap. It will help you to remain alert through the balance of the day and allow your body to better follow its natural rhythms.

Some people take sleep supplements and prescription sleep aids. As I will repeat over and over in this book, I am a strong believer that natural is better. Supplements like melatonin can get you to sleep, that is true, but four hours later they wear off and you wake in the middle of the night facing the choice of taking more drugs or missing more sleep. Further, melatonin can cause an unhealthy spike in blood sugar. Prescription sleeping aids also have side effects. For example, Ambien warns that it can cause problems such as anaphylactic shock, abnormal thinking and behavior changes, decreased inhibitions, hallucinations, complex behaviors such as sleep driving, amnesia, worsening of depression, withdrawal symptoms if stopped, and dangerous interactions with sleep apnea. One of the most extreme cases of overreacting to insomnia is demonstrated by the late singer, Michael Jackson. He literally was dying for a good night's sleep. He directed his personal physician to misuse a powerful sedative to knock him out.

That sedative killed him. I have often said that insomnia is a self-resolving problem. Two or three nights of ordinary insomnia (not caused by some disease process) will result in your natural defenses taking over, and you will sleep long and hard, whether you want to or not. It is best to seek natural solutions to sleep problems, not to take a pill.

In conclusion, sleep is necessary for health and for weight loss. **Make getting a good night's sleep a goal and use a common sense analysis of your individual situation to help you to achieve it.** Occasional insomnia is inevitable for many adults, but will resolve itself in a matter of days. Avoid using drugs to help you to sleep. Seek a natural pattern of rest and it will help you with your health and weight loss.

Seek a positive health loop.

Sleep plays a key role in whether you have a positive or a negative health loop. Imagine the negative. You sleep poorly, so you drink an extra cup of coffee before you leave home. At midmorning, you feel foggy so you reach for the "quick energy" of a donut and a soda. At lunch, you decide to skip the salad you brought from home and go out for a slice of pizza and another soda. In the afternoon, you fear falling asleep in a long meeting, so you help yourself to a free muffin and another cup of coffee. After a long day at work ends, you realize that you have blown your diet. You skip the gym and go home for a frozen pizza, a few beers and top it off with some ice cream in front of the TV. When you go to bed at night, you find your head swimming from all of the caffeine. After you eventually fall asleep, you wake a few hours later with the sheets soaked with sweat from your body burning off the beer. The next morning, you wake up groggy and a little depressed, brew a big pot of extra strong coffee and start the negative health loop over again. If it sounds like I am familiar with this negative loop, it is because I am. Luckily, by becoming simply fit, I have established a healthier loop.

Consider a more positive loop. You block out some extra time for sleep and go to bed early. You sleep through the night uninterrupted and wake before the alarm. You are so ahead of schedule that you cut up some fruit for breakfast and take a short walk around the neighborhood. At work, you feel great and stick to your planned snack of fresh fruit and a healthful salad at lunch. At the afternoon meeting you are on the ball and make a suggestion that the boss praises, boosting your mood. After work, you prepare a healthy stir fry, then head off to the gym where a cute guy or gal asks for advice on how to use the lat pull. You get home exhausted but pleased, hit the sack early like the night before, and fall into a deep sleep quickly and easily.

There is an old saying in education, that nothing breeds success like success. The same saying applies to health. One healthful decision encourages another and pretty soon you start stacking up successes so that their combined value is worth more than the sum of the parts. "Synergy" was an overused term in the 1980's, but it effectively describes the unexpected benefit when all of your health efforts affect your body and mind in a way that is better than the sum of the parts. Look for and maximize opportunities for synergy as you become more fit.

Free heroin.

For many people, the offer of free food is too tempting to pass up. Imagine that you go to the local home improvement store and they are giving away donuts. You know they are bad for you, but you rationalize, "it's free, how can I pass it up?" It is helpful to ask yourself this question, "if they were giving away free heroin, would I take it?" You know that donuts are bad for your health, and re-labeling them as "heroin" or "poison" in your mind will make it easier to pass up the temptation of eating unhealthy free food.

Setting the stage conclusion.

To set the stage for the Simply Fit Diet, stand naked in front of a mirror and take a good look at yourself. Step on the scale daily and record your weight. Set a realistic written weight loss goal and stop by the butcher to see what that extra weight looks like. Before every meal, stand in front of a mirror and raise your shirt, or grab a handful of fat and say, "this is why I need to diet." Finally, make getting a good night's sleep a priority and seek opportunities to establish a positive health loop.

Chapter 4. Dietary Approaches

Dump the junk.

If you have read this far, I will assume that you are one of the almost 70% of Americans who are overweight or obese, but that you have decided to do something about it. The first major dietary step you should take is to **dump the junk**.

When you think of junk food, you likely think of soda, candy and french fries. Foods such as these earn their status as the junk food kings by providing a large helping of calories, with minimal or no nutrition.

For example, a 20-ounce bottle of soda has 250 calories, but little further nutrition. A 32-ounce drink at the convenience store has 390 calories, but a similar dearth of nutrition. On a Summer day, you might even spring for a 64-ounce Double Big Gulp. That mighty serving of junk has 720 calories, 38% of the daily calories a man my size should consume. Although the soda has more than a third of a day's calories, other than carbohydrates and a little bit of salt, it is bereft of nutritional value. The only one who benefits from soda is the soda manufacturer.

Soda is the archetypal junk food, but fruit juices follow close behind. A 20-ounce glass of orange juice has 240 calories, only ten less than a soda, and both have a high glycemic index, meaning the sugar hits your body like a freight train. On the Simply Fit Diet, fruit juices fall into the junk food category and should be eliminated.

Junk calories are not just dangerous because they displace nutritious foods, but also because they physically encourage you to consume more of the same. For a host of complex reasons, the more junk food you eat, the more you crave it. If you think of your fat as "Audrey," she is crying out, "feed me, Seymour," and the food that she demands is junk. Junk serves your fat, and in doing so it actually deprives you of nutrition.

It is not hard to see how Americans can be both overfed and undernourished. Imagine that you get a free airline ticket to get away for a weekend, but your money is tight. You fly to San Diego, stay in a discount motel, and discover there is a McDonald's on the corner. You decide to eat every meal there to save money.

Imagine that you start your day with a Big Breakfast washed down with a McCafe Frappe Mocha. For lunch you have a Premium Crispy Chicken Classic sandwich, along with medium fries and a large cola. For dinner you stick to the classic Big Mac, again with fries and a cola. McDonald's provides a handy online calculator[6] that allows you to total up the calories and nutritional values of its food. For the day, you would have consumed 3,570 calories, enough to add about two pounds per week to your weight if you continued eating this way. Along with the excess calories you would have consumed 154 grams of fat and 740 milligrams of cholesterol, both more than double the recommended intake. However, you would have failed to consume the daily recommended amount of fiber, only 35% of the daily recommended amount of vitamin A, and less than the recommended amounts of vitamin C, calcium and iron. Despite the excess calories in the fast food meals, you would not meet your minimal nutritional needs.

Another example of the same phenomena is found in a simple snack. A four-ounce package of Skittles, a brightly colored sugary candy, has 480 calories, but little nutritional value. For fewer calories than the Skittles, you could eat two apples, two oranges, a banana and ten grapes (Figure 12). But in contrast to the candy's empty carbohydrates, the fruit provides more than the daily requirement of vitamin C, more than half the daily recommended amount of fiber, and significant amounts of calcium, iron, phosphorus, vitamin A, thiamine, and niacin as well as other trace minerals and nutrients.

The government reports that the average American adult gets 19% of his daily calories from solid fats, including fat found in desserts, pizza, cheese, sausage and fried potatoes. Another 16% of the average American's calories come from added sugars, from foods like soda, energy drinks, pancake syrup and candy.[7] Consuming a third of my daily calories in a Double Big Gulp drink may have sounded far fetched in my example a few paragraphs earlier, but in fact **the average American gets 35% of his calories from solid fat and sugar**, both of which are seriously lacking in nutrition. On the other hand, the government reports that 95% of adults under 50 years of age fail to consume recommended amounts of vegetables and 75% of American adults consume less than the recommended amount of fruit every day. Eating junk displaces healthful foods.

Studies show that eating junk food encourages the consumption of more junk food. It is not difficult to imagine why the body keeps asking for more food when on a junk food diet, because it lacks nutrients, despite being fed excess calories. The body asks for more food in an attempt to get the missing nutrients. When you dump the junk, you will not only stop serving Audrey the fattening food she

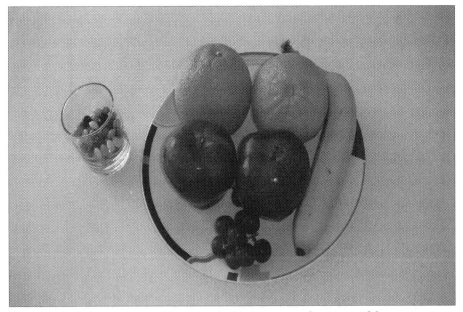

Figure 12. Two snacks. The candy has more calories and less nutrition than the plate of fruit.

desires, you will turn to healthy foods that provide your body with the nutrients it has been missing.

The Simply Fit Diet's definition of junk includes all sodas, cakes, candies, ice cream and fried foods, but goes further. First, all sugar-free sodas and sugar substitutes are included as well. Studies show that, for whatever reason, consuming sugar-free products does not contribute to weight loss, it contributes to weight gain. People who consume these products put on more weight than those who eat the full-sugar products. Why is not clear. Perhaps the sugar substitutes fool the body, which then responds by demanding more sugary foods. Perhaps there is some chemical interaction we do not yet understand. Perhaps the person drinking a sugar-free soda thinks it cancels the calories in the sugar-rich cake consumed at the same time. But the bottom line is that "diet" products lead to weight gain instead of weight loss. Instead of sugar-free soda, drink water. If you like the fizzy treat of soda, you can drink carbonated water like seltzer. Some of the carbonated waters have a twist of lime or lemon in them without artificial sweeteners or sugar. After a day or two of substituting seltzer for soda, you will wonder why the soda was ever important to you.

Second, potatoes are the single food that is most highly correlated with weight gain.[8] This may be because most potatoes are eaten as potato chips or french fries. But it also may be because the highly starchy potato is quickly converted to sugar, a substance that causes a spike in insulin which orders the body to store energy as fat. To be on the safe side, consider potatoes junk and avoid eating them.

My final inclusion in the category of junk is all food with refined grains, plus all foods with added sugar, oil, or salt. Look back at the list of your ten favorite foods on page 30. There are four boxes next to every food listed. The first box is for refined grains, the second for added sugar, the third for added fat or oil, and the last for added salt. For each favorite food, put a check mark in the box that describes its contents. If you are like most people, every single item on your list is a man-made concoction with refined grains or added sugar, oil, or salt. Here's how my list looks:

My Favorite Foods

grains	sugar	fat	salt	
X	X	X	X	1. Pizza
X			X	2. Beer and Pretzels
		X	X	3. Mashed potatoes with butter and sour cream
X		X	X	4. Macaroni and cheese
X		X	X	5. Lasagna
X		X	X	6. Chicken enchiladas
X	X	X	X	7. Chips or crackers and dip
X	X	X	X	8. Pancakes with butter and syrup
X	X	X	X	9. Donuts
X		X	X	10. Pasta with sauce

Trickster foods.

Humans are naturally attracted to sugar, oil and salt. This attraction, in the pre-industrialized world, led us to eat fruits, oily vegetables like avocados, and meat. Modern man has taken this inclination and perverted it by creating foods like donuts (refined grain, sugar and oil, fried in more oil), ice cream (a high-fat dairy product with added sugar and chemicals), pizza (refined grains, usually with added sugar, topped by high-fat dairy, salt, and cured meats). In the name of flavor and profit, industry tailors foods to be high in sugar, oil and salt and reaps the profits. **Sixty-two percent of the foods Americans eat are manufactured with added sugar, oil, or salt** to exploit our natural attraction. The foods that we most frequently consume are not natural. The foods that we like are a man-made exploitation of our natural attraction, but lead us toward disease. These are trickster foods. They trick us into eating things that harm us. What was once an adaptive mechanism has become maladaptive in our obesogenic environment. These man-made foods serve to make Audrey happy, but they lead us to obesity and disease. Unfortunately, **the foods we love make us fat**. The solution is to **limit your consumption of** man-made, trickster foods and stick to natural, single ingredient foods.

Trickster food temples.

Trickster foods are manufactured foods with added sugar, oil, or salt, that appeal to our natural instincts to eat healthy foods, but which have harmful effects. For example, they take a natural attraction to sweets, which would in nature lead us to eat fruit, and instead provide us with milk shakes. Fast food restaurants are trickster food temples. The businesses do not have a goal of making us sick, but they have a goal of making money. The foods that sell best are the foods that appeal to our natural attraction to sugar, oil and salt; but in an exploitive way. A medium apple has 91 calories, 19 grams of sugar and a trace of fat; while a vanilla shake has 530 calories, 63 grams of sugar and 15 grams of fat. However, milk shakes are a staple of fast food restaurants while apples are not. Trickster foods sell the best and make the most money, so fast food restaurants provide them in abundance.

Salt.

Some salt consumption is necessary for human health and salt has been part of human culture for probably as long as human culture has existed. Unlike some people, I am not convinced that salt is evil and must be eliminated at all costs. However, human attraction to salty foods has been exploited by the food industry and most processed foods have incredibly high quantities of salt. The government recommends that healthy young people consume less than 2,300 milligrams of sodium a day, and that people like me who are over 50, or those who are African American, or have diabetes, hypertension or chronic kidney disease consume less than 1,500 mg per day. Half the people in the U.S. fall into the category that should consume less than 1,500 mg per day. The average American consumes 3,400 milligrams per day, and it is not too hard to see how we get there. For example, in the past, I would frequently eat half a frozen pizza for dinner. That serving size contains 3,030 mg of sodium. In one meal, I would consume more than twice the sodium I should consume in a day. Manufactured foods are typically loaded with salt.

Absent a special health reason, I do not think that you need to look at the sodium content of every natural food you eat or to track your daily total. However, you should avoid foods with added sodium such as pizza and most manufactured foods. Just like the foods with added sugar or oil, these are intended to exploit our natural attraction to such foods and effectively trick us into eating foods that hurt our health. Don't go nuts over avoiding salt, but **avoid foods with *added* salt.**

Fat pets.
Another perspective on the dump the junk rule comes from this common sense observation: man is the only animal that manufactures his food. Only man and the animals he feeds (for example, dogs, cats and laboratory rats) get sick from obesity. (A further interesting fact is that the more obese a pet owner, the more likely it is that his pet will be fat.[9]) Animals in the natural world eat whole foods. Animals in the natural world are not threatened by obesity. By avoiding the man-made foods that exploit our natural attraction to sugar, oil, and salt, we can revert to a more natural diet and a more natural weight.

Refined grains.
Grains like wheat grew wild until man began cultivating them about 10,000 years ago. Wheat, the most popular grain, in its unrefined state consists of a hard outer coating called the bran, a pulpy body called the endosperm and a center called the germ. In some ways, it is like an egg with the shell, egg white and yolk. Up until a few hundred years ago, the entire wheat seed was roughly ground to make flour. Modern roller mills allow the miller to separate the wheat germ and bran, and to mill only the endosperm, which creates the tiny particles of refined white flour we most frequently consume today. **About 90% of the nutrients in wheat are removed through the refining process.** In fact, refined wheat flour is so lacking in nutrition that it is "enriched" with man-made chemicals like thiamin, riboflavin, niacin, folic acid and iron, to make up for some of the nutrients that have been removed. However, even when enriched, white flour is not as nutritious as whole wheat flour and lacks the natural fiber of whole wheat flour. The highly refined nature of white flour also makes the chains of sugars dissolve quickly when eaten, resulting in white bread having a higher glycemic

index than a Snickers candy bar. Nonetheless, only 11% of the grains Americans consume are whole grains, and most of these are consumed in breakfast cereals. Refined grains are manufactured foods that lack nutrition and are linked to obesity. Refined grains are junk and should be eliminated from your diet. **Eat only whole grains.**

On the Simply Fit Diet, all foods with refined grains, or added sugar, oil, or salt are junk foods and are to be avoided. Another way of looking at this, is you should eliminate all foods that did not exist before the invention of roller mills that began producing highly refined foods such as white flour. This eliminates most modern convenience foods, but leaves available a whole universe of natural, single ingredient foods like whole grains, vegetables, fruits, nuts, beans, meat and dairy products. For convenience, you may elect to make an exception and allow salad dressings, milks such as almond milk or soy milk, and soy products such as tofu, even if they violate the dump the junk rule.

Dumping the junk may seem a shocking step at first, but take a look at yourself. How has unlimited consumption of man-made junk foods been working for you? Grab a handful of fat. Your answer is there. The foods we have created to appeal to the Audrey within us are subjecting us to an epidemic of obesity and increased risk of diabetes, cardiovascular disease, cancer, and more. Dumping the junk will provide a sound foundation for returning to a natural, healthy weight. Whole foods provide better nutrition than junk food. A bonus of eating single ingredient natural foods will be avoiding the chemicals food manufacturers put in their products for their own convenience. These chemicals are not food and are added for shelf life or palatability. Most of these chemicals are new elements in the food supply and their long term effect is not clear. It is safer to stick with natural foods that have sustained humans for millennia.

Think of your top ten goals, How important are they? Is it more important to have a donut or more important to dance at your daughter's wedding? As one of the almost 70% of Americans who are fat, you should admit that your current strategy is not working. Many people can have an alcoholic drink or two and then walk away. Many people can have a candy or two and then walk away. Some of us cannot. Like an alcoholic, you must admit that the drug you love, junk food, is addictive, and that making a clean break is the best strategy.

And just as friends of alcoholics who are on the wagon do not encourage them to drink, once you quit junk food, you should ask your friends to respect your choice to lead a more healthy life.

Dumping the junk is a key element of the Simply Fit Diet and a rule you should follow for the rest of your life. All of the dietary restrictions that follow the dump the junk rule can later be modified when you reach your weight goal. But for those of us who are subject to weight gain, dumping the junk will be a lifelong strategy. You may say that you are dying for a donut. In fact, that could very well be true. You can choose a life of health or a life of disease. Is the donut really worth the cost? The Simply Fit Diet strategy is to say "no" and to dump the junk.

The world is your watermelon.

What can you eat besides junk? You can eat every whole food in the world. Imagine that all of the food in the world (including the junk) is represented by a big, ripe watermelon. Then picture taking out a large knife and slicing off one end of the watermelon (Figure 13). The end you have cut off represents the junk. Toss it. The remaining food is the food you should eat in the foundation stage of the Simply Fit Diet. There are no other limits on what you eat or how much you eat. You can have oatmeal and fruit for breakfast. You can

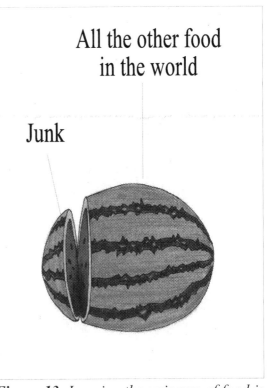

Figure 13. *Imagine the universe of food is represented by a watermelon. Cut off the end representing the junk and toss it. You can eat all the other food in the world.*

have turkey on whole wheat bread for lunch. You can have a big juicy steak with mounds of vegetables for dinner. You can and should have frequent snacks of fresh fruit, vegetables or a hard boiled egg or slice of meat. The world is effectively your oyster (or watermelon). You are simply eliminating the most harmful foods, the foods that encourage you to get fat and the foods that encourage you to eat more of the same. With your daily weigh-ins, you will soon see that Audrey is not happy, and she will begin shrinking to a more manageable size, even with this small step.

Surprisingly, when you break your junk food habit, both the food you desire and the food you enjoy, will change. On the Simply Fit Diet, I enjoy food more than I ever have. However, foods I used to enjoy do not taste the same. For example, I used to eat sweetened yogurt. On the Simply Fit Diet, foods with added sugar are prohibited, so I switched to plain (not vanilla, which has added sugar) yogurt, to which I add fresh fruit. At first, the taste was shockingly bitter, but in a few days it started tasting great. Now, fresh fruit and yogurt is my favorite breakfast. The other day I ordered fruit and yogurt at a restaurant, only to discover that they used sweetened vanilla yogurt. It was disgustingly sweet. I could not finish it. With time, your tastes will change so that foods you used to love become unpalatable and your new diet tastes great. As an added bonus, when you dump the junk you will not only lose weight, but you will be healthier because the natural foods are full of nutrients that are missing from junk foods.

Learn to distinguish cravings from hunger.

If you have been consuming junk food on a regular basis, quitting will lead to cravings. It is important to distinguish cravings from hunger. Cravings make you say, "I could die for a donut." But cravings are limited to one food or class of foods. That is how you can tell a craving is not hunger. If you have a desperate desire for a donut, or alternatively, a candy bar or dish of ice cream, Audrey is demanding that you feed her. Wait the craving out.

Hunger, on the other hand, is much less severe than a craving. Hunger is your body telling you that it is low on fuel and that in the next few hours you should stock up. Hunger is not limited to one food or class of foods. When you are hungry, your body might suggest a donut, but when you say "no," it will say, "how about some grapes?

How about a chicken breast? How about an apple?" **When you are hungry, you desire food, and any food will do.** So ask yourself, will an apple satisfy my desire? If the answer is yes, you are hungry. If the answer is no, you are not really hungry, you are feeling a craving, and waiting until the craving passes will make Audrey shrink and make you healthier. Audrey screams, "feed me." Your body, when hungry, taps you on the shoulder and says, "yo dude, when you get a chance, you might want to rustle up some food." As a matter of survival, hunger is never paralyzing. In the past, you needed the strength to dig some root vegetables or chase down a rabbit. Paralyzing hunger would make that impossible. So if you are facing a paralyzing feeling that you must eat this instance, it is a craving. Go past the cravings and learn to experience the more gentle feeling of hunger. It is natural, and it indicates that your body is taping into its reserves and working the way it should.

Hunger and the hybrid car (learning to live with hunger).

Americans have become so accustomed to easily accessible calories that we almost never feel hunger. As soon as a hint of hunger appears, we head to the pantry or refrigerator, or jump in the car and find a drive-through. However, hunger is a natural part of life. Think of hybrid cars. Hybrid cars are modeled after the way humans use energy. Hybrid cars come equipped with a battery that charges when there is excess energy available, like when going down a hill, and then discharges when the extra energy is needed, like when going up a hill. Similarly, the human body stores excess calories as fat, and draws on those reserves when energy is needed, for example chasing a rabbit for dinner. Hunger is the body's sign that you are drawing down the extra calories, just like the hybrid car indicates it is drawing on its batteries when going up a hill. **I wish I could tell you that you can lose weight and never feel hunger, but that is not true. Hunger is your body's warning light that says you are drawing down stored calories, and you must draw down stored calories to lose weight.** On the Simply Fit Diet, you limit hunger to the evening hours when it is least intrusive, and to night, when your body turns off the hunger warning light to let you sleep. Hunger is a natural feeling. It is not overpowering, it is just your body saying it is dipping into the power reserves. Learn to live with it.

Reverse your cravings.

When you dump the junk, cravings are inevitable. They are usually strongest when your brain is at rest, during break times or during repetitive exercise like walking, swimming, or bicycling. A strategy that makes the craving more bearable and encourages it to pass, is to picture the food that you crave being burned off by your body as the craving occurs. For example, imagine you are on a walk and you crave a donut. You can reverse the craving by saying to yourself that you are now burning off a donut, that you sure ate a lot of donuts in the past and that burning one off is a good thing. Do not starve yourself, eat as much natural, healthy whole food as you desire, but do not give in to cravings for junk food. That would be letting Audrey win. Your goal is to have Audrey shrink and leave. She will not go quietly, but with discipline, she will go in the end and you will have a healthier life.

Bet you can't eat just one. Cheat meals and cheaters.

A few years back a potato chip manufacturer successfully marketed its product with the slogan, "bet you can't eat just one." The slogan was successful because it is true. When you start eating junk, whether for physical or psychological reasons, it is difficult to stop. Some popular diets allow cheat meals and even cheat days. **The Simply Fit Diet does not allow cheat meals or cheat days.** First, one of the proponents of cheat days has been implicated in the sale and use of steroids. It makes sense that a cheater would endorse cheat days. But the physique he sells is not available from healthy living, it is available from drugs. That is not a course I endorse.

Second, there is an addictive component to the foods you crave. Many people scoff at the idea that food can be addictive, but look around you. Addiction is the persistent repetition of a harmful behavior, even though you realize it is hurting you. Recently, I was at the gym and a fellow next to me in the locker room was so heavy, he could barely put on his shoes. He was about my age and obviously sore from carrying at least 100 extra pounds. He neither could reach to the floor nor see his shoes, so he painfully hoisted his foot onto the locker room bench and peered around his stomach to grunt and shove his shoe on. This man was obviously hurting from his weight, yet he slowly grew that big over a number of years. I can only conclude his self-destructive eating habit is evidence of an addictive behavior.

Once you break your physical addiction to foods like donuts and cheesecake, why would you reinsert them into your diet, only to have to break the addiction again? You likely know someone who has had trouble regulating their consumption of alcohol and has resolved this by quitting entirely. Would you suggest that this person start drinking again on certain days or at certain meals? Most assuredly not. If you are overweight, you have demonstrated that you cannot eat as much as you want of everything you crave. You must make certain tradeoffs to maintain a healthy weight. One of these tradeoffs is discontinuing eating foods that make you fat.

Third, it is likely that carb-heavy foods cause a surge in insulin and that surge in insulin directs your body to store fat. The direction to store fat does not disappear after one meal, it lingers for days. In my experience it takes as much as a week to recover from a feast day or a fall off the wagon. The result of a cheat meal or cheat day does not pass in hours, it lingers for days.

Fourth, in this book we have equated eating badly with crashing your car into a concrete barrier. With each crash you cause incremental damage, some of which may not be repairable. Whatever pleasure a donut may give you is unlikely to compensate for losing your leg or other bodily function due to diabetes. If you have a blood glucose meter (available for about $15 at your pharmacy) check your readings after a cheat day. You will likely be shocked to see how high they have risen, often into the range that puts you in danger of diabetes.

Once you attain your weight goal, there will be opportunity to slowly reintroduce favorite foods and to have occasional feasts. But while you are on the path to fitness, in my experience it is far easier to maintain a black or white diet, where some foods are avoided entirely, rather than to blur the lines with cheat meals or cheat days. In my experience, cheat days are for cheaters.

However, if you do fall off the wagon or choose to have a feast day on your reducing diet, it is important that you get back on the wagon as soon as possible. You will compound the damage if, after a fat producing meal, you decide your diet is blown and continue to eat–for example going out for cheesecake. So, if you eat fattening foods, pay close attention to how they taste. It is likely that after having eaten well for a while, they will not taste as good as you imagined. Sweet foods may taste unpleasantly sweet, and salty foods may burn your mouth. After months without pizza, you may be surprised that eating a piece is not a treat at all. Also, it is essential that you step on the scale at your next scheduled weigh-in. Do not skip weighing yourself for a few days, that will only make you more likely to fall off the wagon again. Acknowledge that you made the choice to eat badly and step on the scale and see the damage you have done. Take a deep breath, say, "it is what it is," and record the number. This constant evaluation of your weight and the time it takes you to return to your previous number will make it less likely that you will fall off the wagon again.

The Simply Fit Diet works. One of the reasons it works is because it is a black or white diet. You can eat all of a certain category of food, but none of another. Allowing cheat meals or cheat days undermines this powerful aspect of the diet. Stick to the rules and you will lose. Cheat and you will not.

Foundation conclusion.

This concludes the foundation of the Simply Fit Diet. In summary, make health a matter of life or death before it becomes a matter of life or death. Take a good look at yourself and begin weighing yourself at least once a day. Before meals, lift your shirt and look in the mirror (or grab a handful of fat) and say, "this is why I need to diet." Use common sense to evaluate your sleep habits and strive to get a good night's sleep. Finally, dump the junk. Strive to eat healthy, natural foods and eliminate foods with refined grains, or added sugar, oil, or salt.

The foundation stage of the Simply Fit Diet may result in cravings. Understand that cravings are not hunger. You are free to eat as much healthy, natural food as you desire. Your cravings will pass. After about a week, you should find yourself sleeping better, feeling healthier and free from cravings for your old favorite foods. For some people, these simple steps will be enough to return to a healthy weight. But for me, and most readers, more action is required. At this point you are ready to choose a path to follow in the next stage of the Simply Fit Diet.

Section Three.
CHOOSE A PATH

Chapter 5. The Grain-Free Path

As you choose a path to become simply fit, continue the good habits you established building a foundation for fitness. The most important are to dump the junk, to get a good night's sleep, and to weigh yourself at least daily.

The first path to becoming simply fit is to go grain-free. Most who follow the grain-free path will eat meat and animal products, so if you are or want to be a vegetarian or vegan, you should read this chapter, but follow the food recommendations in the next chapter. But for the majority of readers, the grain-free path will be the easiest, most palatable and most successful.

Please further remember that this section of the book describes a reducing diet. It will help you to quickly lose weight with a minimum of effort and hunger. It is not, however, a diet you must follow for a lifetime. When you reach your weight goal, you will have the opportunity to reincorporate whole grains into your diet.

In Chapter 4, I introduced the concept of the world of food being represented by a watermelon. You have already cut off one end of the watermelon, the section representing junk foods–foods with refined grains, or added sugar, oil, or salt. On the grain-free path, you will cut off the other end of the watermelon, representing all foods containing grain (Figure 14). The remaining portion of the watermelon: all meat, dairy, vegetables, fruits and nuts are available to you in unlimited quantities.

This is a black or white diet. The foods you may eat are crystal clear. For example, if you go to Costco and they are giving out free samples, you do not need to concern yourself with the carb count of the sample, or the fat content of the sample, or the calories of the sample. All you need to ask is, is it made with grain, or does it contain added sugar, oil, or salt? If the answer is yes, you cannot eat it. If the answer is no, have a field day. This simplicity gives the diet its name and makes it easy to follow. The effectiveness of the diet, which you will experience for yourself in the coming weeks, is almost magical.

If you are resistant to the idea of going grain-free, you might point out that government recommendations insist on five, eight or even eleven servings of "healthful whole grains" a day. My first response might be a little rude, but how is that working for you? How is it working for our nation? Since the government starting recommending a low-fat diet featuring multiple servings of "healthy whole grains," obesity has exploded.

A more thoughtful response is to note that the countless studies saying that whole grains are healthy are comparing consuming refined grains with whole grains. I agree, eating whole grains is healthier than eating refined grains. None of the studies compares eating whole grains with eating instead a wide variety of healthy vegetables, fruits, nuts, dairy and animal products. Hopefully, with the rise of grain-free diets, such studies will be conducted in the future, but to my knowledge, none have been conducted yet.

Further, as followers of the grain-free, meat-heavy Atkins diet; as well as followers of the grain-, dairy- and bean-free Paleo diet have been pointing out for decades, grains are a very recent addition to the human diet. Humans have likely been around for 100,000 years and our basic digestive process has been in place for almost a million years. Grains were introduced only about 10,000 years ago. In the history of man,

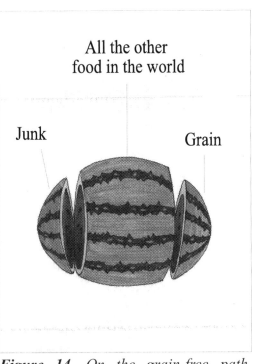

All the other
food in the world

Junk

Grain

Figure 14. On the grain-free path, eliminate the junk and the grain. All the other food in the world is available to you.

74

grain consumption is a very recent experiment. Certainly, for 90% of our history, while our bodies and digestive systems evolved into their current form, grains were absent and unnecessary. They remain unnecessary today. In fact, scientists tell us that **there are no nutrients available from grains that are not available elsewhere**. Grains have no unique nutritional value.

Grains gone wild.
There is general agreement, both among the scientific community and the dictates of common sense, that sugary foods are linked to obesity and that more healthful choices are available. Almost every diet starts by reducing soda, candy and other sugary foods. Scientists developed the glycemic index to measure how fast a food turns to sugar in your blood. The standard score of 100 is assigned to glucose. Granulated table sugar is composed of sucrose (50% glucose and 50% fructose) and has a glycemic index of about 60. Which of the following foods do you think has the highest glycemic index?

- Corn flakes
- White rice
- Bagel
- White bread
- Baked potato
- Table sugar
- Snickers bar

Before I give you the answer, look at the list again and consider which foods you would most likely be willing to consume on a reducing diet. The foods are listed in order of their glycemic index, from highest to lowest. Corn Flakes have the highest glycemic index at 93, white rice is 89, the bagel is 72, white bread follows close behind at 71, the baked potato is 69, table sugar is 60 and the candy bar has the lowest glycemic index at 43. Most people would not eat candy bars on a reducing diet, but might well include rice, potatoes and breakfast cereal. But in fact, the rice, potato and cereal turn to sugar in your blood stream more quickly than the candy bar.

Think of how a bite of plain bread quickly becomes a sugary mass as you chew it. **Grains are starchy foods that are built of**

chains of sugar. The human body quickly disassembles the starch and breaks it into its sugary components so that a bowl of Corn Flakes hits your body faster than table sugar. Most people on diets do not eat table sugar, but they often eat breakfast cereal. Grains are an overlooked source of fat-producing sugar in our diets. Eliminating grains is one of the most effective ways to reduce your weight.

What is a grain?

When most people think of grain, they think of wheat, the most commonly consumed grain in America. However, the list of grains does not end there. Grains include: amaranth, barley, buckwheat, bulgur, corn, couscous, einkorn, millet, oats, quinoa, rice, rye, sorghum, and triticale. Of course, all products made with grain are included as well, including breakfast cereals such as oatmeal, corn flakes, granola and all the other boxed cereals you find in your supermarket. Also included are breads, muffins, baked goods, pop corn, pretzels, crackers, chips, pasta, tortillas, and grits. Do not forget grain-based additives or supplements such as bran or psyllium.

Finally, do not ignore liquid grains–beer being the most common. Hard liquors including whiskey, scotch, vodka and gin are made from grains. Rum is made from molasses or sugar cane and therefore is excluded as part of the junk category. Tequila (made from agave cactus), brandy and cognac (made from wine), hard cider (made from apples) and of course wine made from grapes (but not rice wine) are okay. On this path I do not ask you to stop drinking alcohol (more on this in Chapter 8), just to shift your drinking to a non-grain product.

Beer.

Common sense has long pointed to beer as one of the most fattening beverages. The "beer belly" earned its name through decades of human observation. If you or a loved one is inordinately attached to beer, you might want to ask yourself if your fondness, even addiction, is to the alcohol or the carbohydrates? One way to test this is to replace beer with wine. I like beer. When I replaced beer with wine in my diet, I found that I stopped drinking alcohol altogether. I did not enjoy the wine. In fact, my fondness for beer was for the dose of easily absorbed carbohydrates, not the alcohol. The simple replacement of beer with

---

wine may demonstrate that you crave your favorite beverage for reasons other than the alcohol content.

Adopt a reducing eating pattern.

You should also strive to adopt a balanced eating pattern that assists weight loss. When you dump the junk and avoid grains, you will likely find that you eat more. It may be hard to believe that you can lose weight this way, but you can. You will start losing almost immediately and can expect to lose several pounds the first week, depending on your current weight and dietary habits. As you embark on your weight loss journey, some modification of your eating pattern can help maximize weight loss.

I endorse the old saying which counsels, "**eat breakfast like a king, lunch like a merchant and dinner like a pauper.**" Eating a hearty, healthful breakfast serves many purposes. It breaks your overnight fast and sets you up for a productive day. You can use breakfast as a reward to counter any hunger you may have felt the night before. Breakfast also gives you the energy and nutrition you need for a productive work day. A recent study supports this premise.[10] Two groups of women with metabolic syndrome were put on a 1,400 calorie a day diet for 12 weeks, the only difference was the "breakfast" group had 700 calories at breakfast, 500 at lunch and 200 at dinner; while the "dinner" group had 200 calories at breakfast, 500 at lunch and 700 at dinner. Both groups lost weight. The breakfast group lost 19 pounds and 3.3 inches off their waistlines, while the dinner group lost about 8 pounds and 1.5 inches off their waistlines. The breakfast group also had significantly lower triglyceride, glucose, insulin and ghrelin levels than the dinner group. For example, the dinner group's triglycerides *increased* by 14.6%, while the breakfast group's *decreased* by 33.6%. Simply by eating a bigger breakfast and smaller dinner, the subjects decreased their weight, hunger and risk of diabetes and cardiovascular disease. Without counting calories, the Simply Fit Diet follows a similar pattern, with a big meal at breakfast and a smaller meal at night.

In addition, you should eat snacks at least twice a day: between breakfast and lunch, and lunch and dinner. If you have a busy lifestyle, fruit makes a convenient snack. It needs no refrigeration, contains a reasonable quantity of calories and nutrition, and can be eaten at a desk or on the run. Consider apples, bananas, grapes and other seasonal fruit for snacks, or alternatively nuts, hard-boiled eggs, meat or cheese. Dinner is traditionally the biggest meal of the day, but I recommend that you eat lightly and supplement your entree with a large salad.

I would love to tell you that you can lose weight without ever being hungry, but that is simply not true. When you go into calorie deficit, in effect, you are withdrawing from your fat reserves. Your body lets you know and that feeling is hunger. Because of our jobs, families and multiple responsibilities, the best time to be hungry is at night. On the Simply Fit Diet you should **eat a modest but healthy dinner and then stop eating until breakfast**. No evening snacks are allowed. Especially in the early days of the diet, it is highly likely that by bedtime you will be hungry. It is important to realize that hunger is just your body reporting that it is dipping into your fat reserves. Luckily, the body also has a defense mechanism that turns off hunger when you go to sleep, likely to allow you to sleep. It would be maladaptive for primitive man to be out hunting or gathering at night when most of the large predators hunt as well. But for whatever reason, your hunger in the evening will be short-lived and you will awake and break your fast with a very hearty breakfast.

Strive for variety.

On the Simply Fit Diet, you should strive to eat a wide variety of foods. This can be difficult. I used to eat almost the same thing every day. For example, before becoming simply fit, I liked Grape Nuts cereal for breakfast. I ate it every day. When one box was done, I would have a new one right behind it. The monotony did not bother me.

The problem with eating the same food over and over is that it does not expose you to the wide variety of nutrients, known and unknown, found in different foods. The other side of the coin is that if the food you consume regularly has some dangerous element, for example mercury in fish, you expose yourself to much more of that dangerous element by consistently consuming the same product. Varying the foods you eat, and varying the brands of foods, will expose you to a wider variety of healthful nutrients and avoid over-consumption of harmful elements.

One economical way to vary the foods and brands you eat is to **buy in season and on sale**. Throughout the year, various vegetables and fruits are available in abundance and put on sale. Stock up and eat hardily, because in a week or two, the sale product will change. The same applies to items like yogurt. Instead of choosing a favorite brand, buy the one that is on sale. This not only saves money, but forces variety that can help you to avoid constant consumption of contaminants that may be found in one brand but not another.

Another strategy to force variety is to **run out of your favorite foods**. Let me explain. This is a tough one for me. I always used to have a replacement product sitting on the pantry shelf or in the refrigerator for when the first one ran out. However, running out forces me to find substitute foods. Take apples for example. Apples make a convenient snack. They do not require refrigeration and they can be eaten everywhere. But I tend to get into a rut and eat an apple as part of my morning snack day in and day out. By running out of apples, I force variety. I then choose an orange, grapes, pineapple or some other vegetable or fruit as a snack. For unimaginative cooks like me, running out of certain supplies is a way to force variety into my diet.

Finally, **try at least one new food a week**. The grocery is full of foods that are not on your regular menu. A trip to a whole foods or ethnic grocery store will open up even more opportunities. As you explore the variety of foods available you will increase your exposure to the nutrients they contain and discover flavors you enjoy.

One way to visually evaluate whether you are eating a healthful variety of foods is to look at the colors on your plate. A healthy, natural meal is bursting with color–tomatoes, green peppers, carrots, radishes and so forth. When you see a naturally colorful plate, you can be pretty sure you are getting a healthful meal. To be sure you get plenty of color on your plate, freely supplement your meals with salads. They provide a filling punch of essential nutrients with very few calories. Salads are popular at dinner, but can accompany lunch, breakfast, or serve as a snack. Eat salads freely and frequently.

Stop chasing superfoods.

The term "superfoods" was likely coined by a trade group seeking to increase sales. Blueberries were one of the first foods to claim the title and their sales surged 132%. Other groups sought the same gain.

Sometimes yesterday's unhealthful foods become today's "superfoods." In the past, diet experts warned against consuming too many high-fat nuts. But recently, nut consumption has been correlated with a 20% reduction in overall mortality and a 29% reduction in heart disease among people who ate nuts at least once a day. Further, nut eaters stayed slimmer. The study, conducted by Harvard University,[11] was funded in part by the nut industry and within days, TV advertisements began promoting the health benefits of nuts.

From the other direction, only a few years ago nutrition experts recommended that we eat several servings of fatty fish per week. More recently, studies have shown that for men, high levels of fish oil are positively correlated with prostate cancer and now we are cautioned to eat one or fewer servings of certain fish *per month*. Similarly, antioxidant vitamin pills, once thought to prevent cancer, are now seen as potentially increasing cancer risk.

My point is not to frustrate you with changing definitions of superfoods and dangerous foods. It is impossible to follow each development and science is so limited in its knowledge that today's superfood may be tomorrow's villain and vice versa.

The simple answer is to eat a wide variety of natural, healthful foods. Do not eat the same thing every day. Keep variety in your diet. Buy foods in season and on sale. That will keep an ever-changing variety in your diet. Further, expand your dietary repertoire. Each week, strive to try a new food–maybe daikon radish one week and poblano peppers the next. It will make your diet more interesting and assure that you are exposed to a wide variety of nutrients without over-consuming any single one.

Beware of fattening food combinations.

What do you consider to be the most fattening food? Many people will answer, "ice cream." In the world of common sense, there is broad agreement that foods like ice cream, cheesecake, donuts, cookies, and french fries are uniquely fattening. This common wisdom is likely drawn from how eating these foods shows up on the scale almost immediately.

Some will say that these foods are fattening merely because they are rich in calories. This may be true, but it is also a very real possibility that certain food combinations are more fattening than their mere caloric content dictates. There is growing evidence that there is a qualitative difference among calories and that certain foods cause a surge in blood sugar, resulting in a surge in insulin, and that insulin tells your body to store fat. So in the case of ice cream, the added sugar sets up the insulin surge. The body then has an order to store fat, and the ice cream provides fat aplenty. A two-cup bowl of rocky road ice cream provides 84 grams of carbohydrates and 20 grams of fat (including 12 grams of saturated fat, 60% of the recommended daily value on a 2,000 calorie diet), a formula for weight gain that likely exceeds its abundant 560 calories. Consider your ten favorite foods. Most, if not all of them, are a combination of carbohydrates and fat. Most, if not all of them, are man-made trickster foods with quantities of carbohydrates and fat not found in nature. Look at my list:

1. Pizza
2. Beer and pretzels
3. Mashed potatoes with butter and sour cream
4. Macaroni and cheese
5. Lasagna
6. Chicken enchiladas
7. Chips or crackers and dip
8. Pancakes with butter and syrup
9. Donuts
10. Pasta with sauce

Every item on the list is high in carbohydrates. The only item without significant added fat is the beer and pretzels. All of the others have a combination of carbs and fat that encourage weight gain. Take a look at your list on page 30. How does it stack up? While you have the list out, please do this: in the title "My Favorites," cross out the word "My," and write in "Audrey's." It is about time that you recognize that the foods you thought you loved are really supporting your fat. They make Audrey happy but over time they make you sick. At least on a rational basis, you can start to see these foods as man-made toxic combinations that hurt your health.

Point out the poison.

Think of your ten favorite foods. Typically, if you saw a picture of a favorite food, for example a brownie, you would say, "yum." The alternative to skipping the yummy food would then seem like deprivation. But the foods you listed are man-made concoctions that twist a healthy drive for sweets (like fruit) into an unnatural diet that makes you fat and can lead to diabetes, cardiovascular disease and other ailments. Because you are a person who is inclined to get fat, brownies are not a healthful treat, they are effectively poison for you. If you see a TV ad for brownies and you say out loud, "poison," you will begin to change your thinking. You will start to realize that brownies are not an innocent treat, they are bad for your health.

For practice, pick up a color advertisement from a local grocery store. In your mind, or out loud, call all the whole foods advertised "food." All of the manufactured foods and foods containing refined grains or added sugar, oil, or salt should be labeled "poison." As you go through the ad you will find that the "poison" advertised far outweighs the "food." In fact, around certain holidays I find that entire advertisements are made of pictures of poison. Is it any wonder that so many Americans are fat?

If certain food combinations are more fattening than their mere calories dictate, it explains why some very similar meals have different effects. For example, a seven-ounce steak at a popular restaurant provides 280 calories, 15 grams of fat and 1 gram of carbohydrates. When eaten with a side of steamed broccoli, there is very little carbohydrate directing your body to store fat. However, when eaten with a side of mashed potatoes, the order for fat storage goes out and the meal may be far more fattening than the sum of its calories. Similarly, a meal with carbohydrates but without fat may be less fattening than one that combines both. For example, a pita bread filled with garden salad has 37 grams of carbohydrate, but very little fat. The same pita bread stuffed with a cheeseburger has an abundant supply of fat to be stored when the body receives the order to do so from insulin.

The grain-free path of Simply Fit Diet eliminates most foods with added fat, but has no restrictions on foods with natural fat content. For example, meat, cheese and dairy products are all allowed. However, the diet broadly restricts the carbohydrates that typically accompany these fatty foods. The Simply Fit Diet allows you to have steak with broccoli, but prohibits steak with mashed potatoes. This path's limitation on carbohydrate consumption may be why it works so well.

Mete out the meat.

Here's a quiz for you, which former President said he ate meat only, "as a condiment to the vegetables which constitute my principal diet?" Your most likely guess is Bill Clinton. After all, Clinton, having had two heart surgeries, has become vegan (consuming no meat or animal products and no eggs or dairy), a move he credits with saving his life. The visibly slimmer Clinton now weighs 175 pounds, the first time he has been at that weight since age 13. The quote is actually from one of our most famous Presidents, Thomas Jefferson, who for health reasons elected to make plants the center of his diet. Jefferson lived to age 83, quite a feat considering the less developed state of public health and medical care that existed when he died in 1826.

My recommendation is much less severe than the one followed by Jefferson or Clinton. At this stage in Simply Fit Diet, I recommend that you **eat one meal with no animal products at least once every six meals—once every other day**. Lunch is a great time to introduce this strategy. A salad with fresh greens, avocados, a variety of vegetables and a sprinkling of nuts, needs nothing else.

Americans eat animal products at virtually every meal. You may protest that you do not have animal products at breakfast, but do you use milk, cheese, cream in your coffee or manufactured foods that include animal byproducts? Probably so. Skipping animal products at least once every six meals will give your body a break from the constant presence of high-fat, high-protein animals. If such products are a source of artificial hormones or antibiotics, it will give you a break from these as well. Further, shaking up your dietary options will encourage you to try new foods—a stir fry with daikon radish or tofu can be just as tasty as one with meat, but will give your body exposure to a new source of nutrition.

Further, American portions of meat are huge when compared to those consumed by people around the world. I was lucky enough to live in Asia for a while. At the inexpensive street-side stands I frequented, the dishes were entirely vegetarian until the very end of their preparation, when the proprietor would go to a case, remove a little bit of meat, cut off three or four paper thin slices and then put them on top of the vegetables.

If the Asian approach seems extreme to you, don't worry, I am not insisting that you adopt it. However, do consider that American servings of meat are large. If you prepare your meals for two or more, **consider splitting a serving of meat between the two people**. Half a standard steak or half a plump chicken breast, when supplemented with salad and vegetables, will make a hearty, healthy and satisfying meal, but can also assist you in trimming your weight painlessly. You can still have a juicy steak, just top it with mushrooms, onions and chilli, and serve it with a colorful side salad. Food should be appetizing, colorful and fun. You do not need to suffer on the Simply Fit Diet.

What do you eat?

A day on the grain-free path is not a day of deprivation. In case you are having a hard time imagining what to eat, here is my typical grain-free diet day. I start out with a big bowl of fresh-cut seasonal fruit, mixed with plain, full-fat yogurt. For a morning snack, I have a banana and an apple. At lunch I have a vegan salad based on prewashed organic greens bought at a big box store, supplemented with seasonal vegetables including avocado, with a sprinkle of sliced almonds and some dried seaweed. For an afternoon snack I will have another banana and some cashews (a tasty combination) as well as another seasonal fruit. For dinner I have a stir fry with seasonal vegetables, some daikon radish, as well as a small serving of meat–perhaps shrimp, chicken or beef. On the Simply Fit Diet, you will find that food tastes better than ever and that you enjoy it in larger quantities than in days gone by. You should eat as much as you desire to feel full, just remember, after dinner, don't eat any more. It is good to get a little hungry before bed, it helps you to wake up with the goal of eating a hearty breakfast and starting out on another full day of healthful eating.

Avoid drinking your calories.

Throughout most of man's history, water was the primary beverage. Fruit juices, wine and beer are recent inventions–only in the past several thousand years. Coca-Cola arrived on the scene in 1886,

Gatorade started in 1965, and energy drinks, the most recent high calorie fad, have only become a significant force in the past decade. When compared to the hundreds of thousands of years that humans have been around, most caloric beverages have only been available for the blink of an eye. Therefore, it would not be surprising that the body tends to ignore beverage calories.

Scientific studies support this premise. In one study, students were allowed to eat as much pizza as they wanted, accompanied by no beverage, a non-caloric beverage, or a caloric beverage such as milk, soda, or orange juice. *The students ate the same amount of food, whether or not they consumed a beverage, and felt just as full, whether or not the beverage had calories.* However, when the beverage had calories, these calories were added to the meal–the student's bodies did not seem to count the liquid calories as food calories.[12]

Although the pizza-eating study found that milk acted like soda or juice, other studies find milk the exception to the body ignoring liquid calories. This makes sense. We are designed to thrive on human milk, and cows' milk is a similar substitute. In some studies, milk is the single beverage that the body seems to acknowledge and therefore reduce the consumption of other foods.

Government statistics reveal that the average American adult drinks 400 calories a day in the form of regular soda, energy and sports drinks, alcoholic beverages, milk, 100% fruit juice and fruit drinks, in that order. Caloric beverages constitute 21% of all calories consumed by the average American. Even when the 2.9% of calories (about 64 calories a day) the average American drinks in the form of milk are excluded, **if the average American would replace the non-milk caloric beverages with natural zero calorie drinks and not replace those drinks with other calories, he could lose 35 pounds a year!**

To make this concept work on the Simply Fit Diet, eliminate all non-milk caloric beverages. You can still drink plain coffee and tea, water and carbonated water. If the body doesn't count caloric beverages, then eliminating them will not make a difference in your hunger, but will speed your weight loss.

Skip the low-fat products.

I, like so many Americans, fell victim to the advice that low-fat products were more healthy than full-fat products. In my early 20's, I gave up full-fat milk and started drinking skim milk. Now, more than 30 years later, research shows that for both children and adults, low-fat products are correlated with obesity while the full-fat products result in lower weight and better health. My efforts to be more healthy likely resulted in my being less healthy.

On the Simply Fit Diet, I encourage you to eat natural, whole foods. Full-fat milk, although far from what comes from a cow's udders, is a more natural product than non-fat milk. In fact, if carbohydrates make you fat, this helps explain why reduced-fat products do not work. For example, a cup of full-fat milk has more calories than non-fat, but non-fat milk, having been modified by man, has more carbs. Whole milk gets about 30% of its calories from carbohydrates while non-fat milk gets about 56% of its calories from carbohydrates. And that is if you would consume the same liquid quantity of each product. If full-fat milk is more filling, it is quite possible that you would consume less of the full-fat product. If you consumed 100 calories of full-fat milk, compared with 100 calories of non-fat milk, the differential in carbohydrate content is amplified. The 100 calorie glass of full-fat milk has about 5.5 grams of carbs, while the non-fat has 14 grams.

Reduced-fat products do not make you thin and may make you fat. On the Simply Fit Diet, there is no reason to consume reduced-fat products, enjoy the more natural full-fat products.

Monitor the scale and work with the program.

Everyone is different and not all foods affect us the same way. Modify the Simply Fit Diet to work best for you. For example, some people are adversely affected by beans, nuts, wine, or soup. Notice if your weight increases consistently after eating certain foods. If it does, limit your consumption of that food. You can certainly defeat any diet, including the Simply Fit Diet, if you say it does not work and quit. Instead of seeking defeat, seek success by modifying the diet to fit your individual constitution.

Changes to expect.

If you follow this diet exactly, the changes you experience will be sharp and almost immediate. Because you are weighing yourself daily, you will be able to track your weight loss closely. Depending on how much weight you need to lose, you will lose several pounds the first week. You will not maintain this pace, but it will encourage you to keep trying.

After a few days of living without grain, you will also notice that you sleep better. This sounds like a bold, unsupported claim, but it is true. The reason for this is unclear. Perhaps the lower levels of insulin allow deeper sleep or perhaps grain acts as an irritant to the body. But for whatever reason, this diet enhances sleep and sleep enhances weight loss. It is part of the positive feedback loop.

Further, if you have lived a certain number of years and feel sore in the morning, your soreness will improve. The improvement will not be startling, but after a few days you will notice a bit less soreness. The way I thought about the decreased soreness is this, it is not miraculous, but if the improvement came in a pill, I would pay for it and take it. Some people would explain this by saying that grain causes inflamation and eliminating grain avoids the inflammation. Others might say that sleeping better improves soreness. Another explanation could be that losing weight reduces the strain on your muscles and joints, or that better nutrition makes the body work more efficiently. Why soreness improves on this diet it not clear, but it is a welcome side effect for the aging body.

Also, it is highly likely that your mood will improve. It could be because you are sleeping better. Or maybe it is because your body is getting better nutrition and starting to work efficiently, or maybe your outlook improves simply because you are starting to see weight loss results. But for whatever reason it occurs, it is welcome.

The first place you will lose weight is from the umbrella of fat that sits inside your rib cage. This is good. First, losing this weight will significantly decrease your chance of diabetes and other diseases. Scientists say that a 7% weight loss is all it takes, and losing that 7% will come surprisingly quickly. Second, losing weight from your internal stores will likely result in a decrease in your pants or dress size. This clear and early success will encourage you to continue with the diet.

Later weight loss will come from your external fat stores, starting in the areas furthest from your belly and draining down. Fat often disappears from the face early, resulting in recognition of your weight loss efforts by your family and peers. The last place you lose weight is usually the first place you put it on, often the belly. This will provide you with a final push into smaller clothes before you reach your weight loss goal.

In the early days of the diet, it is important to continue to look at yourself in the mirror before meals, but as you begin to lose weight, instead of saying, "this is why I need to diet," start saying, "I am doing well, but I can do better." Eventually you will reach the point where you are pleased with what you see and you will discontinue the before-meal ritual.

At the start of the diet, you made a trip to the butcher shop to see a tangible representation of the weight you need to lose. Pretty soon, you will have lost several pounds. Now when you go to the butcher shop, find a package of meat equal to your weight loss. Even a single pound is meaningful, and ten pounds is really impressive. Pick up the meat and think about how much better you feel not carrying that weight around, every step and every minute of the day. Think how much easier it is for your body to provide nutrients and waste disposal to the slimmer you. This step may seem silly, but it is both a useful reward and a useful preventive measure. As a preventive measure, if you are tempted to break your diet, think again about that ten-pound package of meat. Ask yourself if you really want to stick that weight back on your body. After you consider the consequences, it is likely that you will decide that no food, no matter how attractive, is worth putting back on the weight you fought so hard to lose.

As your weight loss continues, you will likely need to buy new clothes. Think of the waist size or dress size you wore when you were at your target weight. Between now and then you will likely need to resize several times. I recommend that you buy a pair of pants or other outfit in the next smaller size, even if it does not yet fit. It will motivate you to make it fit, and reward you when it does. It will also amaze you when you have to pack it away (or give it away) when it becomes too big. As I lost weight, I moved progressively down in waist size from size 36 to size 30. It was incredibly rewarding to watch the sizes shrink.

As the weight disappears, you will notice some markers that you had forgotten existed. You may start to see your clavicle, or collar bone. Later the latisimus dorsi (angel's wings on your back) may appear. Finally, you should begin to see your ribs–when was the last time you saw those? Next, the saddle bags on your sides will shrink, along with your belly. The final place you will lose weight is the first place you put it on, for many men the belly, and for women, often the belly or hips. As you reach your weight goal, you will become trim for the first time in years.

As you close in on your target weight, beware the advice of people who say you have lost too much. They may be well meaning, but think of it, the majority of Americans are overweight or obese, your friend may be saying "too much" in relationship to everyone else. Thank the friend for his or her concern, but stick to your own counsel. If you are worried about losing too much, visit your doctor and seek his or her advice.

You will likely have reminded yourself that you have been on a reducing diet, not a lifelong diet. You have been maintaining a deficit of about 500 calories a day. As you reach your weight goal, you will have the opportunity to either eat more and/or to eat differently. This decision is a delicate one, and is discussed more in Chapter 11.

Why does this diet work?

There is a great divide among nutrition experts as to whether losing weight is simply a matter of limiting calorie intake, a position I will call calories in/calories out, and those who believe there are qualitative differences among the foods we eat, that some foods actually make us fatter than others. As a preliminary matter, it does not really matter why this diet works, as long as it works.

The calories in/calories out crowd could point to the list of the most frequent sources of calories for adult Americans. Out of the 28 foods on that list, this path of the Simply Fit Diet eliminates 16 (Figure 15). Although the Simply Fit Diet encourages you to eat as much healthful food as you desire, the calories in/calories out crowd would argue that with less access, you are getting fewer calories and therefore are losing weight.

The qualitative calories theory is different. This theory says that the foods you eat affect you differently and some foods are more inclined to make you fat, while others are not. In its simplest form, this theory says that high carbohydrate foods cause a spike in blood sugar (recall the high glycemic values of grains and sugars). The spike in blood sugar leads to your body producing more insulin. Insulin tells your body to store fat. The high carbohydrate foods, according to this theory, will make you fatter than other foods, even if you consume the same number of calories of each. The grain-free path of the Simply Fit Diet broadly limits carbohydrate intake.

Of course, there could be a completely different reason why this diet works. Perhaps because you eat large quantities of natural foods on the Simply Fit Diet, you get more fiber and the fiber aids weight loss. Or maybe some undiscovered phytonutrient in the many plants you consume has a similar effect. Maybe there is an unknown factor X that makes the diet work. Or perhaps the constant monitoring and goal setting (daily weigh-ins and thrice daily reminders of why you need to lose weight) make it work. Likely it is a combination of factors that makes the Simply Fit Diet successful. The scientific consensus is that the best diet is the one that works. The Simply Fit Diet works. It does not really matter why.

Grain-based desserts
Yeast breads
Chicken and chicken mixed dishes
Soda/energy/sports drinks
Pizza
Alcoholic beverages
Pasta and pasta dishes
Mexican mixed dishes
Beef and beef mixed dishes
Dairy desserts
Potato/corn/other chips
Burgers
Reduced-fat milk
Regular cheese
Ready-to-eat cereals
Sausage, franks, bacon, and ribs
Fried white potatoes
Candy
Nuts/seeds and nut/seed mixed dishes
Eggs and egg mixed dishes
Rice and rice mixed dishes
Fruit drinks
Whole milk
Quickbreads
Soups
Other white potatoes
Other fish and fish mixed dishes
Crackers

Figure 15. The grain-free path of the Simply Fit Diet eliminates 16 of the 28 foods Americans most commonly consume.

Summary.

So far, you have built the foundation for the Simply Fit Diet by deciding to make losing weight a matter of life or death before it becomes a matter of life or death. You have taken careful stock of your current health and weight and you have begun weighing yourself on at least a daily basis. You have gone to the butcher shop and taken a look at a quantity of meat that approximates the amount of weight you need to lose and you have considered how carrying around that extra weight affects your health. Before every meal, you have gone to a mirror and raised up your shirt, or you have grabbed a handful of fat, and you have told yourself, "this is why I need to diet." Finally, you have taken a slice off the watermelon of available foods by eliminating all foods with refined grains, or added sugar, oil, or salt.

On the grain-free path, you have eliminated all grains from your diet. You will eat hearty servings of vegetables, fruits, nuts, meat and dairy. You will eat whole foods and avoid man-made low-fat and diet products. You will incorporate healthy snacks, often vegetables or fruit, into your routine. You will have broken your addiction to junk food and grains. You will know the difference between cravings and hunger, and as your diet improves, your cravings will disappear. You will eat a big breakfast and a small dinner. You will choose to be hungry at night, and you will accept hunger as a natural consequence of weight loss.

You will strive to try at least one new food a week and you will seek to eat a wide variety of healthful foods. You will have at least one in six meals free from animal products, and you will reduce meat portions at other meals and instead incorporate hearty servings of vegetables.

Your weight will decline steadily, at first at a fast rate, but as time passes, at a slow and sustainable pace. Each week you will stop by the butcher shop and grab a package of fatty meat equivalent to the weight you have lost. When your friends ask you if eating only one donut will really hurt, you will think about the weight lost represented by the meat, and you will answer, "yes it will." You will need to buy new clothes, and your friends and coworkers will ask you about your weight loss.

But most important, you will feel better. You will sleep surprisingly well and wake with much less soreness than in years past. You will have more energy for exercise and your mood will improve.

As you pass your weight loss milestones, your likelihood of disease will decline. You will be well on your way to becoming simply fit.

Chapter 6. The Vegan Path

The Simply Fit Diet promotes itself as accommodating the desires of the most committed carnivore as well as the most virtuous vegan. The previous chapter described one path to fitness, a path that a larger number of readers will likely find easier than the path described in this chapter. However, both paths have their merits, and features of each are likely found in the most healthful diet. If you skipped the previous chapter, please go back and read it. Strategies described in that chapter should be used on the vegan path, including:

- Adopt a reducing eating pattern: eat breakfast like a king, lunch like a merchant and dinner like a pauper. Be hungry at night.
- Strive for variety in your food, including buying in season and on sale. Try a new food weekly.
- Beware of fattening food combinations.
- Avoid drinking your calories.

Do you know any fat vegans?

The most prominent feature of the path described in this chapter is the substantial elimination of animal products from your diet. A person who does not eat animal products (no meat, no fowl, no fish, no eggs, and no dairy) is known as a vegan. The question at the start of this section is, "do you know any fat vegans?" You likely know some fat vegetarians. Vegetarians do not eat meat, but generally eat dairy products and eggs. A vegetarian could comfortably chow down on a spinach and mushroom pizza dripping with cheese. A vegan would not. Some religious groups promote vegetarianism, like Hindus. But when you see photos of crowds in Hindu areas, you often see overweight people. Vegetarianism does not automatically lead to a trim figure, but veganism does.

On this path, I do not ask you to give up animal products completely, although you may if you choose. Rather, I ask that you only eat animal products, including eggs, dairy products, fish, fowl and meats, once every six meals or less. Further, I ask that you continue to "dump the junk," as described in Chapter 4. That means no manufactured foods with added sugar, oil, or salt.

The grain-free path eliminated all grains, but on the vegan path you may eat whole grains with the exception of wheat. That means you can have a hearty bowl of oatmeal with fruit for breakfast. Your lunchtime salad might include quinoa, and your evening stir fry can be served over a bed of brown rice. Using the watermelon analogy, you have already cut off one end of the watermelon representing junk food. On this path, cut off the other end of the watermelon representing animal products and take off one more slice representing wheat (Figure 16). All of the remaining food in the world can be your diet on this path.

Giving up animal products sounds quite radical to many people. Meat is integrated into American culture. For men, meat and masculinity are nearly synonymous. A generation ago, Daddy was the one who would, "bring home the bacon." For many men, the best dish they can cook is meat on the barbeque. To think of life without meat is radical. However, there are many reasons to consider eliminating animal products from your

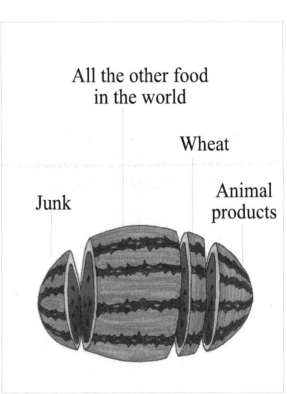

Figure 16. *On the vegan path, eliminate junk, animal products and wheat. All the other food in the world will be your diet.*

diet. The first is because the animals we kill and eat are sentient beings who feel pain. Some people choose not to eat animals because they do not want to kill them. Another is that animals are on top of the food chain. They take enormous resources to grow and they produce enormous waste when killed. It would be easier to feed all of the hungry people in the world if so many resources were not dedicated to producing extremely resource-rich animal products. But these philosophical reasons to become vegan are beyond the scope of this book. This book is about losing weight and achieving fitness and a mostly vegan diet helps to achieve that goal.

First, studies show that vegans are lighter and healthier than the general population. Compared to omnivores, vegans have lower rates of coronary heart disease, hypertension, diabetes and cancer. Vegans are less likely to be obese and more likely to live longer than the general population.

Second, there is growing evidence that consumption of red meat and animal products is correlated with an increased risk of cancer and circulatory diseases. The National Institutes of Health says, "past research has tied red meat to increased risks of diabetes, cardiovascular disease and certain cancers. The studies have also pointed to an elevated risk of mortality from red meat intake."[13]

T. Colin Chapman, in his book *The China Study*, describes studies of mice exposed to carcinogens where their risk of developing cancer could be turned on and off *not* by the amount of carcinogen exposure, but by the amount of animal protein in their diet. Incredibly, mice with low animal protein intake had no cancer, even when exposed to the same quantity of carcinogens as the animal protein-eating mice who developed cancer. Scientists cannot ethically experiment with people the way they do with mice, but in a huge study of regions with diverse diets in China, Chapman demonstrated that the areas with the highest animal protein consumption also had the highest levels of disease.

In the prior chapter, I described the advantage of eating a wide variety of foods. Veganism multiplies this advantage. First, fats have about nine calories per gram. Carbohydrates only have about four calories per gram. On a vegan diet, you will displace the calorie-dense fats found in meat, cheese, and other dairy products with lower calorie options. Therefore, to get the same number of calories, you will need to eat more food. For example, a 7-ounce steak at a popular chain restaurant has 280 calories and provides 34 grams of protein. You can get just as much protein by eating broccoli, but it will take a 44 ounce serving, and that serving will have 170 calories, still less than the steak. To equal the calories of the steak, you would need to eat about nine cups (72 ounces) of broccoli. As you can see, you need to consume more food to meet your nutrition needs on a vegan diet.

Of course, humans like variety. Your diet will not consist solely of broccoli. You will naturally seek out and consume a wider variety of foods, especially vegetables and fruits, when you are on a vegan diet. This wide variety of vegetables and fruits will provide your body with large quantities of the healthful nutrients plants provide, both known and unknown.

You will also note that I have asked you to eliminate wheat while on the reducing phase of this path. There is growing evidence that wheat is the most fattening grain and for many people may have harmful effects. For an exploration of reasons why wheat may be bad for you, check out William Davis' book, *Wheat Belly*. But I am not so concerned about the reasons, just the results. Elimination of wheat helps with weight loss. One explanation of why eliminating wheat helps with weight loss is that wheat is the most commonly consumed grain in America–it is in almost everything. Eliminating wheat while on a reducing diet may help you to lose weight because you will simply have fewer eating options. An alternate explanation is that wheat causes a surge in insulin which tells the body to store fat. Eliminating wheat may lead to weight loss by lowering insulin levels. Please remember that beer is made with wheat and is restricted on this path. You may choose to drink wine or other non-wheat based alcoholic beverages on this path.

The thought of starting a vegan diet is probably more difficult than actually doing it. The first time I went on a vegan diet was in response to my brother losing his leg due to diabetes. I read *Dr. Neal Barnard's Program for Reversing Diabetes* and thought I would give his method a try. At first, I said I would go a week without meat. But later I decided I would go one day without meat. Finally, the night before starting the vegan diet, I retreated to agreeing to breakfast without animal products. I consider myself a relatively open-minded, non-macho American man, but I found meat and animal products to be deeply ingrained in my lifestyle. However, once I skipped animal products for one meal, I found the results positive. I gave them up almost completely. I did not die. I did not pass out from lack of energy. And although I started eating more frequently than I had before, and eating more volume than I had before, my weight dropped steadily until it reached a healthy level. If you try the vegan path, you will find that animal products are *not* necessary for health or energy, and that you obtain a more pleasant, lean-burning energy from vegetables, grains and fruits.

The Eden diet.

Whether you think the Bible is the work of God, or an interesting historical document, it has enormous impact on our culture. The Bible starts with man and woman living in the Garden of Eden, and their diet is vegan. They eat no meat or other animal products. Genesis 1:29 recounts that God created man and said, "I give you every seed-bearing plant on the face of the whole earth and every tree that has fruit with seed in it. They will be yours for food." On the surface, meat and animal products are imbedded in our consciousness and culture. But when you dig a little deeper, so is veganism. If you believe that the Bible is the word of God, you should also consider that the ideal diet described in the Bible is a vegan diet.

To juice or not to juice.

The wide availability of high speed juicers and the recent popularity of films like Joe Cross' *Fat, Sick and Nearly Dead*, have made juicing popular. Juicing effectively takes a vegan diet and liquefies it. A frustration with juicing is that a single fruit or vegetable produces only a dribble of juice, so a large mass of plants is required to make a meal. Further, the abundant fiber the body would normally obtain from the vegetation goes into the garbage. Personally, I prefer to "juice" my vegetables with my teeth and to get the full benefit of nature's goodness from the food I eat. On balance, I see juicing as a bit of a gimmick, but if it is a gimmick that gets people to eat healthy food and lose weight, I see no harm to it on a short term basis.

Protein and vitamin B-12 on the vegan path.

People unfamiliar with a vegan diet may wonder if it provides adequate protein. The government recommends that women get 46 grams of protein a day and men get 56. Plant products like tofu, beans, and nuts provide plentiful protein. For example, a cup of cooked soy beans has more than 30 grams of protein, a cup of lentils has 18 grams of protein and a four-ounce handful of cashews has 20 grams of protein. If you consumed all of these in a day, you would have 68 grams of protein. It is not difficult to put together a healthy diet with more than enough vegan protein.

Vitamin B-12 is another matter. Animal products are rich in vitamin B-12, but non-fortified plant products lack this essential nutrient. The government recommends that people over age 14 get 2.4 micrograms of vitamin B-12 a day. As a preliminary matter, your body's store of vitamin B-12 will last for months before experiencing a deficiency, so a short time on the vegan path should cause no harm. Further, on the vegan path you may consume animal products once every six meals. Occasionally eating three ounces of cooked clams would give you about 84 micrograms of vitamin B-12.

However, both vegans and about 30% of people over the age of 50 are at risk of a vitamin B-12 deficiency. Artificial sources of vitamin B-12 can help. Eight ounces of fortified soy milk provides three micrograms of vitamin B-12 and two tablespoons of fortified yeast provides 7.8 micrograms. Many fortified breakfast cereals provide generous doses of vitamin B-12, although it is hard to find a cereal without added sugar. You could also take a vitamin B-12 supplement. If you follow a mostly or completely vegan diet you should research the issue of vitamin B-12 requirements and meet with your doctor to establish whether supplementation is appropriate for you.

Vegan cave men?

Proponents of the paleo lifestyle will likely gleefully ask, "have you ever heard of a vegan caveman?" The answer is, "not really." However, I would ask, "have you ever heard of a caveman who drove his leather-interior 4x4 truck with one-touch down power windows to the drive-through and traded a piece of paper representing ten minutes of his time for a day's worth of calories?" The answer to this question is, "certainly not." Paleo diets are currently popular and are easily accommodated on the no-grain path. However, paleo diets, vegan diets, and almost all diets, for that matter, are artificial restrictions of the dangerous abundance of food we have created in recent years. A more important question than, "did cave men do it?" is, "does it work and is it healthy?" A vegan diet both works toward weight reduction and is healthy.

Why does the vegan path work?

Following the vegan path on the Simply Fit Diet leads to consistent weight loss, even though you will probably be eating more volume and more frequently than on your previous diet. Vegan advocates point out that an animal-free diet contains much less fat than a carnivorous diet. If consuming fat makes you fat, the vegan path provides a solution. Further, obtaining almost all of your nutrition from plants forces you to eat a large volume and variety of plants. Plants are more nutritionally rich than animal products and those nutrients may make you healthier and help you to lose weight. Alternatively, eliminating almost all animal products and wheat products limits the foods that are available to you. This may result in your consuming fewer calories, providing an explanation palatable to the calories in/calories out crowd. And most probably, it is a combination of these factors. However, the important thing is not why it works, but that it works. Following the vegan path will result in steady weight loss, and as long as you stay on the path, you will reach your weight goal.

Vegan path conclusion.

When you plan a trip, there is usually more than one path to your goal. The same applies to weight loss. Both the grain-free path and the vegan path will lead to steady, sustainable weight loss and help you to improve your health and lower your chances of disease. The changes you can expect on the vegan path are the same as the ones described for the grain-free path starting on page 86.

Chapter 7. Exercise: You Gotta Move

For 99% of man's existence, he has been in a life or death struggle to get enough food to survive. Our bodies have evolved to prevail in this struggle. However, over the past few hundred years, we have achieved overwhelming success. We have made calories cheap, easy and always available. At the same time, we have virtually eliminated the physical struggle to obtain these calories. We face a circumstance our bodies are ill equipped to handle–the horn of plenty described in Chapter 1. This horn of plenty creates a new threat to our health, the threat of too much food and too little activity. Most diets, the Simply Fit Diet included, artificially limit food and increase activity. The great substance of this book has been dedicated to diet because diet is the largest component of weight loss. This section however, is dedicated to another essential component of fitness, physical activity.

Beyond a certain age, it is virtually impossible to maintain fitness with exercise alone. Heaven knows I tried. I like to think of myself as not too dim a man, but it wasn't until I was 50 years old that I recognized both intellectually and emotionally that what I put in my mouth is the largest component of the fitness equation. At least three-quarters of weight loss comes from diet. The greatest substance of weight loss work occurs in the kitchen and dining room, not in the gym. However, as a nation, we seem to spend three-quarters of our effort on exercise.

On the other hand, that does not mean that exercise can be ignored. Exercise helps to lower your risk of every single disease that is related to obesity, including heart disease, stroke, diabetes, depression, and cancer. Exercise helps to prevent and control obesity. Exercise is a necessary part of the fitness equation. I like to think of it this way, imagine you have a garden hose that won't quite reach a tree you want to water. If you compress the hose on one side, the water will go further, but not far enough. Only by compressing the hose on both sides can you make the water reach your goal. Similarly, even though diet is the most important part of the fitness equation, you will unlikely meet your fitness goal unless you compress both sides of the horn of plenty, on one side with diet and the other with exercise (Figure 17).

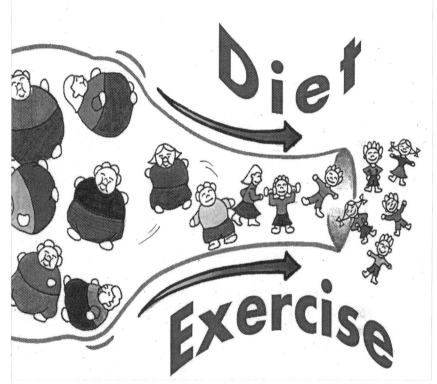

Figure 17. *To most effectively become fit, you must squeeze the horn of plenty on both sides.*

The National Weight Control Registry[14] tracks people who have lost over 30 pounds and kept the weight off for more than one year. The members have lost an average of 66 pounds. Not surprisingly, 98% of the members modified their food intake to lose weight. But tellingly, **94% also increased their level of physical activity, with the most common activity being walking. Members exercise about one hour per day.** The largest database of successful dieters demonstrates that both diet and exercise are important and that about an hour of exercise a day is desirable.

Statistics about Americans' level of physical activity are pitiful. The American government recommends that adults get at least 150 minutes of moderate activity or 75 minutes of vigorous activity a week. For maximum benefit, the government recommends 300 minutes of moderate activity or 150 minutes of vigorous activity per week. We fail badly. Only 42.6% of women and 52.1% of men meet the *minimum* recommended level of exercise. Twenty-four percent of Americans report they engaged in absolutely no exercise in the prior month.

For children, the government recommends 60 minutes of exercise per day, every day. By the time kids reach age 15, only 31% meet this level of activity on weekdays and 17% on weekends. Tellingly, however, the average child spends 7.5 hours per day in front of a screen (TV, computer, tablet, cell phone, or entertainment media like video games). Adults spend 8.5 hours per day in front of a screen.

Our lives are full of labor-saving devices. When you think about it, even your chair is one of them. The great majority of our forebearers did not have comfortable chairs, they sat on the floor. Nowadays, a test the doctor can use for fitness is how easily you can go from a standing position to sitting on the floor and back up again.[15] Give it a try. Do you rise easily or do you have to use your hands and knees as you struggle off the floor? Modern Americans are far less active than our bodies are designed to be. The developer of the test says that it is a strong predictor of mortality in middle-aged and older people. The more you need to use your hands or knees and the more unsteady you are, the more likely it is that you will die prematurely. In the study, those who performed best were 21% less likely to die, while those using the most support (using more than one hand or knee on the way down and more than one hand or knee on the way up) were five times more likely to die. After you try this test and understand its implications, you should feel more motivated to exercise. Physical activity is natural and essential to both weight loss and overall health. **On the Simply Fit Diet you should strive to do an hour of physical activity a day.**

Activity choices.

Walking is America's most popular activity and probably the simplest activity available. You need no special clothes or equipment, no set time or location, and you do not need to pay fees to walk. You can just put down the book, head outdoors and participate in one of the most natural and essential activities available. Walking can be brisk or leisurely. It can be a solo or group activity. It can be during the day, at night, or on a break from work. It can be for minutes or for hours. Unless your health is seriously compromised, there is no excuse for not walking. Those who are unaccustomed to exercise will want to start out slowly. Go for a distance that is comfortable and enjoy your walk. Simply add a little more distance every time you try. Even if you only add one or two steps a day, soon you will be able to walk for distances you once thought unimaginable. Do not let embarrassment about your weight or appearance stop you from getting out and exercising. You are doing this for yourself, not for an audience. Make health your number one priority, and as you lose weight, your embarrassment will turn to pride.

A natural extension of walking is running. We are not designed to hop in cars and travel to drive-through windows in air-conditioned comfort. That is a product of our inactive society. We are designed to pick berries, dig roots and chase rabbits. Running is part of our natural activity. Just like walking, running can be engaged in on a very small scale. When I started on my path to fitness, I had an injured back and three or four paces running was all I could handle. But with each step I grew stronger. To me, there is something completely natural and harmonious about running, something healing and healthful and different from what walking brings. Perhaps it is that the heart beats faster, the lungs open wider, and the legs stretch longer. Perhaps the body secretes and releases necessary hormones when you run. I do not know, but running, even for a very short distance like six steps, is a natural, healthful human activity that I recommend for those who are fit enough to participate in it safely.

However, the best exercise is one that you will do. Everyone is different. Looking back to the activities you liked as a child or young adult can often help you to identify an enjoyable physical activity. Did you like to bicycle as a youth? Inexpensive bikes are available at yard sales and big box stores, why not get one and try riding again? Did you like to swim? Most localities have public pools, and many private clubs have pools open all day. Jump in and see how it feels. How about team sports? Were you a volleyball player or ice skater? There may be leagues you can join to reconnect with your old interests. Countless opportunities for physical activity exist. As a matter of health, you should pursue them. If you are at a total loss of what exercise to try, here in rank order are the most popular ones in the U.S. according to the Census Bureau:

Walking
Fishing
Exercising with equipment
Camping
Swimming
Bowling
Working out at a club
Bicycling
Weight lifting
Hiking
Aerobics
Running/jogging
Billiards
Hunting
Target shooting
Basketball
Boating
Golf

Yoga
Skiing/snowboarding
Soccer
Table tennis
Backpacking
Softball
Baseball
Tennis
Volleyball
Football
Skateboarding
Mountain biking
Scooter riding
Roller skating
Archery
Paintball games
Water skiing
Ice hockey

Time for exercise.

In our hectic world, many people complain that they have no time for exercise. For most, the time is available, it is just not a priority. For example, the average American adult spends 8.5 hours per day in screen time. Anyone who within the last week has watched their favorite show, played a video game, checked Facebook or sent a non-work text message, has time to exercise. Reducing screen time and increasing physical activity will make you more fit.

Stress.

Stress has an enormously negative impact on health. It increases stress hormones, speeds aging and changes the way our bodies function. Stress relief can be found in quiet moments, keeping journals, meditation and in exercise. Screen time tends to increase stress. Time spent in nature or with friends or animals reduces stress. Many people see exercise time as time to put on earphones, hook up to the cell phone and continue the electronic bombardment. Instead of keeping the steady drumbeat of music and technology, why not enjoy your time in nature *without* electronic enhancement? You can then "multitask" your exercise time by adding electronics-free stress reduction to your exercise routine.

Exercise conclusion.

Although the majority of weight loss comes from diet, exercise is an indispensable part of the fitness equation. An optimal level of activity is at least one hour a day. There are countless forms of exercise, but the best exercise is one you will do. Sometimes looking back to your youth will help you to rediscover the joy of bicycling, swimming, skiing or some other long forgotten activity. Absent a connection to a particular form of exercise, America's most popular sport, walking, is a great way to start. Find time for exercise by reducing screen time, and you will soon see gains in your overall fitness.

Chapter 8. Bad Habits

Most people have bad habits. Two of the most common dietary bad habits are excessive consumption of caffeine and alcohol. Most diet books give you little leeway in dealing with these habits. The authors dismissively declare that you should stop drinking alcohol and coffee on the first day of the diet and leave it at that. If only it were that simple. These habits can be deeply ingrained and if the diet insists that you give them up, the diet is more likely to end up in the trash, rather than your habit.

I will not ask you to give up your bad habits on the first day of the Simply Fit Diet. However, I will ask you to reduce them. The standard of how much caffeine or alcohol is too much is a very personal one. One or two glasses of either is likely no problem. Four or more glasses of alcohol or eight or more cups of coffee likely is a problem. The approach I suggest is that at the start of the Simply Fit Diet you **reduce your consumption of alcohol and caffeine by one third**. For example, if you drink three mugs of coffee a day, reduce the quantity to two. If you drink three alcoholic beverages at night, cut back to two.

Additionally, consider altering your pattern of consumption. Try to stop drinking coffee by noon every day. This has two benefits. First, you give your body time to process the chemicals in your system, allowing as many as 20 hours without caffeine. Second, by giving your body extra time to process the caffeine before bed, it is likely that you will sleep better, with all the health benefits that brings. Further, if you sleep better, you are less likely to want an extra cup of coffee in the morning.

With alcohol, consider drinking earlier in the evening and stopping well before bedtime. If you usually have a drink with dinner, and one or two afterwards, consider switching to a before-dinner drink, and wrap up the drinking with your meal. If one of your goals is to become a little tipsy, drinking before your meal can probably get you tipsy on less. More important, you will let the alcohol wear off a bit more before bedtime, allowing you to sleep more deeply. The reduction in drinking will also cut calories, leading to a more steady weight loss.

Are bad habits good?

In Woody Allen's movie *Sleeper*, a health food store owner from 1973 is frozen and brought back to life in 2173. In the comedy, science in the future world has demonstrated that many of his healthy techniques were wrong, and many of the things he thought were bad have been proven healthy. A look at current research can make you feel like Woody Allen's character in *Sleeper*. Sunshine, once thought to be a cancer causing factor to be avoided at all costs, is now considered essential to health. Sunscreen, which we were told to slather on in great quantities, may not reduce the incidence of skin cancer. Alcohol, once thought to be bad in any quantity, may be a health tonic, and coffee, almost always seen as a bad habit, may be a useful antioxidant and dietary aide.

Alcohol.

Let me say first, that I have seen alcohol destroy the lives of friends and relatives. I like to drink and I have had some of the best times of my life while drinking. However, if I could wave a magic wand that would wipe away all of the alcohol in the world, I would. Unbridled consumption of alcohol has caused incredible pain and damage. If you do not drink, I would never recommend that you start. However, if you do drink, there is growing evidence that moderate alcohol consumption can be good for your health.

Researchers report a "U" shaped relationship between alcohol consumption and health. That is, it is healthful up to a certain limit, and then becomes harmful. Alcohol consumption, be it beer, wine or hard liquor, has been found in limited quantities to improve your health and longevity, including reducing the chances of arthritis, cancer, dementia (including Alzheimer's disease), diabetes, enlarged prostate, and stroke.[16] Some researchers say that moderate alcohol consumption provides a 40-60% reduction in coronary heart disease, and the benefit of moderate drinking exceeds the benefit of exercise on heart health. A meta-analysis shows a 30% reduction in the risk of diabetes associated with moderate alcohol consumption.

Specifically how much alcohol is good for you is unclear. The American government says one drink a day for women and two drinks a day for men is healthful. Other countries specify different limits, for example Canada allows up to two drinks a day for women and three drinks a day for men, the United Kingdom allows up to three drinks a day for women and four drinks a day for men.[17]

What's a "drink" of alcohol?

The U.S. Government says a standard drink has 14 grams of alcohol. So how much wine is that? If a bottle of wine has 25 ounces, or 5 drinks, a glass has 5 ounces. If that liquid is 12% alcohol, a glass of wine would have 14 grams of alcohol and equal one drink. However, if you only get four glasses out of your bottle of wine, your glass of the same wine would have 6.25 ounces and 17.5 grams of alcohol. Looking through my wine rack, most wines have an alcohol content of 13.5% and the highest is 14%. That 14% wine in a 6.25 ounce glass would have 20.4 grams of alcohol, or slightly less than one and a half standard drinks.

With beer, 12 ounces at 5% alcohol constitutes a standard 14 grams of alcohol drink. But at the local pub, beers are typically served in 16 ounce pints, resulting in 18.7 grams of alcohol in a pint. Make that draft a popular IPA at 7.5% alcohol and your pint has 28 grams of alcohol, exactly *twice* the alcohol in a standard issue government drink. The percentage of alcohol in your glass and the size of that glass has a real impact on calculating the risk or benefit of that drink.

Another consideration relating to alcohol consumption is that alcohol has about seven calories per gram–almost double that of carbohydrates (four calories per gram) and almost as much as fat (nine calories per gram). You should carefully consider if you want to spend your calories on alcohol instead of a hearty salad or a piece of fruit.

Further, the body schedules alcohol for priority processing. That is why, if you go to bed soon after consuming a few drinks, you will likely wake up a few hours later feeling hot and sweaty. The body burns off the alcohol calories first, leaving it to store the remaining food calories you have eaten. This can lead to weight gain, particularly if you supplement your alcohol with unhealthy food.

Also, the alcoholic beverages you may consume are basically fermented fruit juices, and the Simply Fit Diet categorizes fruit juices as junk. Further, there is the very real possibility that the body does not count beverages as food. That is, a glass of wine with your meal does not make you feel more full and you will eat the same amount as if you had consumed water. If that is true, the alcohol you consume is simply added calories, and the calories are mostly from sugar and alcohol.

Whether you drink or not is a complex adult decision. **The best course is to eliminate alcoholic beverages completely while you are reducing to your weight goal, and then consider adding them back when you reach your weight goal.** At that point, you can control your diet carefully and see if you experience any weight gain from consuming the beverages.

Drinking to remember.

My Mother died of Alzheimer's. It was a terrible disease that started when she was about my age. It slowly robbed her of her memory and eventually control of her body functions until she regressed to an infantile state before dying. Having observed this, I am highly motivated to avoid Alzheimer's disease and dementia. Some scientists say that alcohol consumption reduces the risk of dementia. A British meta-analysis concluded that moderate alcohol consumption is correlated to a reduced risk of Alzheimer's disease by 32% and dementia by 38%.[18] Other studies find a risk reduction of up to 80%.[19] Of course, correlation and causation are not the same thing. Umbrella use is correlated with rain, but it does not cause rain. However, even the conservative USDA Dietary Guidelines conclude, "[m]oderate evidence suggests that compared to non-drinkers, individuals who drink moderately have a slower cognitive decline with age." The hope that moderate alcohol consumption lessens the risk of dementia led me to add a glass of wine to my dinner, despite the added calories. However, that dietary change led to steady weight gain for me and I have eliminated wine from my diet.

The alcohol/caffeine connection.

Bad habits sometimes come in pairs. Anyone with some life experience has had a friend or loved one who drank a bit too much at night and compensated with an extra large dose of caffeine to get to work in the morning. The same person might go to bed at night, be unable to sleep from all the caffeine, and have an extra alcoholic beverage as a "nightcap," to help knock him or her out to get ready for another day of work. The up and down cycling of alcohol and caffeine is a common crutch and can throw off the body's delicate balance. It is good to watch for it in your life and the life of people you care about. Bad habits are easy to repeat, but when they are replaced with healthy habits, they too can become routine. Health is a habit that should be encouraged.

Caffeine.

Caffeine is another substance about which the science has changed, and if you have not been keeping up with the changes, the latest information may make you feel like Woody Allen in *Sleeper*, being told that what you thought was bad for you is now good for you. The government has not gone as far as saying that drinking coffee is good for you, but it says that moderate coffee consumption is not harmful.

A few years back, it was widely assumed that caffeine consumption was a negative, or at best a neutral habit. Caffeine *does* disturb sleep and elevate your heart rate and blood pressure. However, the most recent studies claim that caffeine, like alcohol, has a U-shaped effect on health, up to a point, it may be good for you, and beyond a certain point, it is bad for you. Caffeine has been shown to reduce the risk of gallstones, liver cancer, dementia, diabetes and to improve alertness and attention. For diabetes, a Dutch study concluded that drinking seven cups of coffee a day reduced the risk of diabetes by 50%, compared to those who drank two or fewer cups a day.[20] A meta-analysis found a reduction of the risk of diabetes of 5-10% per cup of coffee consumed a day, up to 6-8 cups.[21] For people with diabetes or pre-diabetes, it would likely be worthwhile to review the research on coffee consumption with your doctor for a recommendation of whether coffee might reduce your risk of diabetes.

For some time now, dieters have realized that caffeine, particularly a cup of black coffee, not only quells hunger, but seems to encourage weight loss. There is growing support for this. A recent study provided 12 overweight subjects with pills containing green coffee extract. Over 22 weeks, they lost an average of over 17 pounds each, with no significant change to their diets.[22]

It is probably not a good idea to go out and start drinking coffee as a dietary aid, however, if you are a coffee drinker, it may not be necessary to quit. Further, with this knowledge in hand, coffee makes a good substitute treat. For example, if your friends go out for an afternoon slice of cheesecake, you can forgo the cake, but enjoy the camaraderie and a nice cup of premium coffee.

Be careful with the cup.

Coffee consumption is usually measured in "cups." Cooks know that a "cup" is a term of art, meaning eight fluid ounces. But a lot of people like me refer to their coffee mug as a cup. My coffee mug, however, holds 16 fluid ounces. So even on days I have a single mug of coffee, I consume two cups. In judging the best dose of coffee for health effects, be sure to know how many cups fit into your mug.

Further, the quantity of caffeine in a cup varies from brand to brand. Starbucks coffee has about twice the caffeine of Folgers coffee. So a 16-ounce medium sized Starbucks "grande" coffee could have as much caffeine as four measured cups of standard coffee.

Treats.

If you are overweight, it is likely that you use food as a reward. On the Simply Fit Diet, you should strive to find non-food rewards. There's nothing I enjoy more than watching a sunset while drinking a cold beer. However, it is not too far a step to watch the same sunset with some sparkling water or herbal tea. Similarly, I used to enjoy passing milestones with a dinner out. On the Simply Fit Diet, I eat out much less frequently–it is easier to get a wide range of healthfully prepared natural foods at home. But the same money that would be spent on dinner can be used for other treats–for example, as you lose weight, you will need new clothes. The price of a dinner celebration can

111

buy a new shirt, dress, or other wardrobe items to help celebrate the new you that is emerging.

Convenience stores: the addiction stop.

Pretty much everything sold at convenience stores caters to the addictions of the customers. I used to stop by for coffee in the morning (an addiction) and watch customers pick up a few small bottles of booze, a soda in which to pour the liquor, and some chewing gum or cigarettes to cover the smell. The aisles are full of cases of donuts, heat-and-eat burritos and hot dogs spinning on a grill. Alongside the beer, wine and liquor are colorful cases of soda, sports drinks, and the newest addiction, energy drinks–potent combinations of caffeine, sugar and other stimulants marketed to the young. At the cash register, you can buy a few dollars of lottery dreams–less likely to pay off than getting struck by lightening. On the Simply Fit Diet, convenience stores are good places to avoid, and if you find yourself buying a product typically featured at a convenience store, you should ask yourself if you are feeding an addiction.

Bad habits conclusion.

As an adult, you make complex choices about your conduct, including bad habits. As a preliminary matter, caffeine and alcohol consumption may not be as bad for you as you once presumed. However, both are addictive and can have negative effects on your life. You should try to reduce your bad habits by one-third. Further, you should carefully evaluate how these habits fit into your lifestyle and affect your health. Especially when you are on a reducing diet, it is probably better to eliminate alcohol consumption until your body reaches a healthy weight. Then, especially with any addiction broken, you can decide if it belongs in your life and to what degree.

Chapter 9. Chemicals, Chemicals, Chemicals: Supplements and Over the Counter Drugs

Nutritional supplements.

If you haven't been following the latest developments in nutritional supplement science, you might again feel like Woody Allen in *Sleeper*, being told that what you once thought was good for you is now bad for you.

I freely admit, I have been duped. For years, I took multivitamin/mineral pills. Now studies show that even these simple pills have no benefit and may cause harm. Even the medical profession is coming around on this issue. In late 2013, the journal *Annals of Internal Medicine* published a series of vitamin studies accompanied by an editorial entitled, "enough is enough: stop wasting money on vitamin and mineral supplements." They said, "[beta]-carotene, vitamin E, and possibly high doses of vitamin A supplements are harmful. Other antioxidants, folic acid and B vitamins, and multivitamin and mineral supplements are ineffective for preventing mortality or morbidity due to major chronic diseases . . . we believe that the case is closed–supplementing the diet of well-nourished adults with (most) mineral or vitamin supplements has no clear benefit and might even be harmful."[23] For the average healthy adult, vitamins are unnecessary. However, for women who are or may become pregnant, consultation with a physician is appropriate before making a decision about vitamins and minerals.

Fortified or enriched foods.

Vitamins and minerals not only come in pills, they can be added to food. Did you ever wonder how so many breakfast cereals provide exactly 25% of the recommended dose of a host of nutrients? It is because the cereal effectively contains a multivitamin/mineral pill mixed in with the grain. Manufacturers generally use the term "fortified" or "enriched" on the product's label to alert you that chemicals have been added. The government reports that commonly fortified products include:

- Rice and other whole cereal grains
- Flours, cornmeal, bread and pasta
- Breakfast cereals
- Milk and milk products like yogurt and soy milk
- Fats and oils like margarine
- Salt, monosodium glutamate, sugar and sauces
- Tea and fruit juices

If you want to avoid chemicals in your food, watch out for fortified or enriched products. Further, if you feel the need to supplement your diet with a multivitamin/mineral pill as 67% of Americans do, understand that you may be duplicating the pill's effect if you consume fortified or enriched foods.

It seems like every day there is a new report that chemicals we once thought were good for us are actually bad for us. Did you use antibacterial soap? I did. But now the government says that plain soap is just as effective as antibacterial soap, and that the common antibacterial ingredient triclosan (also found in Colgate's Total toothpaste) may have a harmful effect on human hormones. How about mouthwash? A new study concludes that mouthwashes containing the chemical chlorhexidine kill useful bacteria in the mouth that help to control blood pressure. Simply using mouthwash resulted in increased blood pressure in the subjects that raised their risk of stroke by 10% and heart disease by 7%.[24] How about foot powder? Harmless, right? But by killing off useful flora on the foot, it could do more harm than good. Sunscreen? Some of the chemicals used in sunscreen may be hazardous to your health, some studies show that sunscreen use is correlated with *higher* rates of skin cancer, and sunscreen use has been implicated in creating unhealthy reductions in vitamin D metabolism.

It seems the more we learn, the more we learn to question chemical use. I am not suggesting that you do not use foot powder or mouthwash, but I am suggesting that you only use chemicals based on a need, not on a fear. So, use foot powder only if you have athlete's foot, instead of in case you get it. Take aspirin because you are sore, not because you fear you may become sore. Take vitamins based on a medically identified need instead of taking them, "just in case." The more we learn, the more we learn that chemicals are not harmless and sometimes they have unintended consequences.

Do you know more than God (or Mother Nature)?

Whether man is the product of divine creation or natural selection, we are extremely complex beings built to function in a natural, un-supplemented world. Outside of when there is a specific disease process or medical need, man's meddling with the human system has done more harm than good. If you have a specific medical need that calls for nutritional supplements or medications, you should follow medical advice. However, a multibillion dollar industry exists to make you *think* that you need supplements. Humans love the idea of a magic pill and the industry is ready to take your money and provide you with one. However, absent a medical need, the pill is at best a waste of money and at worst harmful. When it comes to nutritional supplements, I suggest this maxim, "when in doubt, take the natural route." A wide range of natural, healthful foods provides all the nutrition that a normal, healthy adult needs.

Use your free annual check up to ease your mind.

The Affordable Care Act, also known as ObamaCare, requires health plans to provide a free annual checkup and related laboratory tests. Take advantage of this free information when you start your diet and get medical advice. Ask your doctor to conduct tests to see if you are lacking any nutrient, or if your position in life puts you at risk of nutritional deficiencies. Absent medical advice to take supplements, get your nutrition from food, not chemicals.

> **Vegans, people over 50, and vitamin B-12.**
>
> Both vegans and people over 50 have some risk of being low on vitamin B-12. Following the Simply Fit Diet vegan path, you can have animal products once every six meals or so, therefore vitamin B-12 deficiency is unlikely. Further, only about 30% of people over 50 are at risk of vitamin B-12 deficiency, so taking it just in case may be unnecessary. Once again, I recommend having a blood test to see if this deficiency exists, instead of automatically taking chemicals.

Over the counter drugs.

The human body maintains a delicate balance that can be thrown off by consuming chemicals. Like many, I formerly consumed over the counter drugs without much thought. I figured that if they are available without medical supervision, they could not be too strong or dangerous. However, that is not true.

Personally, I became dependant upon omeprazole, sold as Prilosec. This drug is used to treat an acid stomach. The instructions say not to take it for more than two weeks. I asked my doctor about this and he said it was just an exculpatory warning and that most everyone took it on a regular basis. So I did. However, over time the drug became less and less effective. I also developed increasingly painful arthritis in an ankle I had hurt long ago. After some research I learned that Prilosec is implicated in limiting calcium absorption and can cause the exact type of arthritis symptoms I was suffering. It was quite difficult to taper off and quit Prilosec. I felt like I had a stomach full of hydrochloric acid, but after I quit, my arthritis symptoms lessened significantly.

Another over the counter drug generally labeled safe is melatonin. I have taken it on occasion to sleep better. However, for me and for many other users, melatonin causes a spike in blood sugar. I did not know this and was never warned of it. I only discovered it when I began testing my blood sugar on some mornings and found an inexplicable spike after taking the drug. Of course, I have discontinued it.

As time passes and I accumulate life experience, I more clearly see the wisdom of avoiding drugs and chemicals wherever possible. The human body has an enormous ability to heal and regulate itself.

Man's chemical interventions into this area often do more harm than good. When in doubt, take the natural route.

Food chemicals.

Chemicals are often added to manufactured foods for the convenience of the manufacturer, to give the food longer shelf life or to increase its marketability to consumers. Check out a few food labels on the shelves of a convenience store. You will likely be surprised by the list of chemicals. On the Simply Fit Diet you will get the greatest substance of your nutrition from single ingredient whole foods. A side effect of the Simply Fit Diet is that you will substantially reduce your consumption of chemicals added to manufactured foods.

Chemicals conclusion.

In conclusion, when it comes to taking nutritional supplements, over the counter drugs and medicinal chemicals, you should take them based on a medically identified need, not based on hope, fear, or habit. If you need to take drugs, go ahead and take them. But **when in doubt, take the natural route**.

Section Four.
STAY SIMPLY FIT

Chapter 10. Merging the Paths

The Simply Fit Diet differs from most diets by offering two dietary paths. Both paths share a foundation of dumping the junk and focusing on single ingredient natural foods. The grain-free path allows broad consumption of meat and animal products, while the vegan path eliminates animal products almost entirely. It is highly likely that if you have followed one path or the other, you will favor it and want to stay on it. That's fine. However, as this book comes to a close, I have a few more suggestions.

Weight loss is a slow process, akin to steering an ocean liner. However, weight loss is easily observable on your weight chart. You know your diet is working when the numbers go down.

Choosing the most healthy diet possible, however, is not as easy. Answers to questions like, "does meat consumption increase cancer risk?" and, "does wine consumption decrease the risk of dementia?" are not provided in weeks or months on a weight chart. Answers to these questions will take years and the issues may not be clearly resolved in our lifetimes. Choosing the most healthy long term diet is based, to a great degree, on feelings, hunches, guesses and faith. The recommendations I make in this chapter are completely optional. They do, however, reflect my opinion of the most healthy diet.

There are definite indications that consuming large quantities of meat and animal products is positively correlated with getting cancer and heart disease, and conversely eating large quantities of vegetables and fruits is negatively correlated with cancer and heart disease, perhaps because of some protective effect of the vegetables and fruits. This correlation disappears when animal products constitute less than 10% of the total calories consumed.

I have used both the vegan path and the grain-free path to maintain a healthy weight. In my estimation, the grain-free path is the easiest, but on it, it is easy to slip into consuming a large quantity of animal products that may be harmful in the long term.

Similarly, the vegan path is effective, although I must admit as a pure vegan, with my high level of physical activity, I felt a bit low on energy and my muscle mass decreased alarmingly. For me, a pure vegan diet did not provide all of the nutrients I felt I needed for optimal function.

My solution is to merge the grain-free and vegan paths. I eat animal products only once every three to six meals, and then as part of a meal–a bit of meat in a stir fry or served over a bed of lettuce, or some yogurt with my morning fruit. For me this incorporates the best of both paths, the cancer and heart disease avoidance of the vegan path plus the extra energy of the grain-free path. Whether you choose to stick with one path or to merge them as I have done, is strictly up to how you think and feel. The main goal of the Simply Fit Diet is attaining a healthy weight. You can do that on either path.

Chapter 11. The End of the Path and the Second Most Dangerous Decision

I have repeatedly reminded you that the Simply Fit Diet paths are a reducing diet and that you do not need to stay on forever. But when you reach your weight goal, you face a very hazardous time–almost as hazardous as the day you started the diet. As many as **90% of typical dieters regain the weight they have lost**. The Simply Fit Diet's lifetime plan of weight monitoring will help you to avoid the weight gain that plagues many dieters. Still, when you reach your numeric goal and look at yourself in the mirror and find yourself amazed and satisfied with your reflection, it is very easy to revert to old habits. I strongly encourage you *not* to go back to your old eating habits. That will result in an amazingly fast rocket trip back to your old weight or even higher. It is important to *slowly* introduce foods you have eliminated and to carefully evaluate how they affect your weight.

Here is an example of what I am talking about. On the grain-free path, creating interesting breakfasts can be challenging. After you reach your weight goal, you may wish to reintroduce oatmeal to your morning meal. My suggestion is that you have it one morning and then do not repeat the meal for three days. Carefully evaluate how the new food affects you and track whether it leads to weight increase. If you tolerate it well, keep it on your menu and move on to another food–for example adding some brown rice to your evening stir fry. Once again, only do it once every three days and carefully evaluate its effect. You get the idea. Do not make wholesale changes to your diet or it could quickly get out of hand. Decide what you want to eat, experimentally add a bit of it to your diet, and continue to carefully monitor your weight.

Audrey's ghost.

Earlier in the book I asked you to imagine that your fat is like a foreign invader that has taken root in your body and is screaming, "feed me." When you complete the Simply Fit Diet, Audrey will be gone. You will be fit and trim. But Audrey's ghost remains. Her vestigial roots will call out quietly, "a little pizza won't hurt." When you are fit, it is easy to listen to Audrey and try to eat like everyone else. But you are not like everyone else. Remember, you have a problem with weight and a little carelessness will pile the weight on quickly. You must be good on your diet to the point of being near-perfect. Do not give in to Audrey. Remember **the price of fitness is constant vigilance**.

It is highly likely you will start to gain weight. Set a limit of how much weight gain you will accept without taking action–perhaps ten pounds. If you exceed this amount, strip away the added foods, give your body a chance to adjust to the change, and use the tools you have learned to return to your weight goal. Then, more slowly and carefully, add foods back into your diet.

Remember, the price of fitness is constant vigilance. You have made a long journey from fat to fit, and it is worth the effort it takes to maintain your current state of fitness. Do not stop recording your weight, the action of recording your weight will help you to maintain your weight loss. Also, remember that fat accumulates again in the opposite pattern in which you lost it. So if your belly is the last place to become trim, monitor it for increased fat deposits. The mirror as well as the scale should be a tool in the constant vigilance it takes to maintain fitness.

You can and will reach your weight goal. But this is a critical time. Do not go back to old habits. Slowly experiment with excluded foods and pull back when weight increases. Congratulations on becoming simply fit.

Chapter 12. Summary of The Simply Fit Diet

We live in a virtual horn of plenty, where fattening foods and inactivity result in almost 70% of adult Americans being overweight or obese. Being fat is dangerous, increasing your risk of a host of diseases, including diabetes, cardiovascular disease and dementia. On a systemic basis, the solution is simple, we need to squeeze the horn of plenty with healthy foods and increased activity so that we return to a healthy weight. But on a personal basis, the issue is much more complex. Losing weight takes effort. To motivate you to make that effort, I recommend making fitness a matter of life or death before it becomes a matter of life or death

To build a foundation for the Simply Fit Diet you should take a good look at yourself. Really. Stand naked in front of a mirror and evaluate where you are. Further, step on the scale. Weigh yourself today and every day for the rest of your life. Monitoring your weight is an essential step to becoming simply fit. Set a reasonable weight goal based on yourself, not people you see on TV. Write that weight goal down. Remind yourself of your weight goal before every meal by standing in front of a mirror and lifting up your shirt, or by grabbing a handful of fat and saying, "this is why I need to diet." Understand that a good night's sleep is important to weight loss. Make sleeping well a personal goal and use common sense to help you to reach that goal.

Acknowledge that you have a weight problem and give up eating junk, for today and forever. Define "junk" as all foods with refined grains, or added sugar, oil, or salt. Also eliminate potatoes, diet and low-fat products. Instead, focus on eating natural, whole foods. If you imagine the universe of food as a watermelon, cut off one end representing junk food and permanently discard it.

To help you return to a healthful weight, you will need to go on a reducing diet. The Simply Fit Diet provides two paths, the first path is to stop eating grains and grain products. That means no amaranth, barley, buckwheat, bulgur, corn, couscous, einkorn, millet, oats, quinoa, rice, rye, sorghum, triticale, or wheat. If you picture the watermelon representing the universe of food again, cut off one end of the watermelon representing junk and the other end of the watermelon representing grain. Toss them. All of the rest of the food in the world is available to you on this path of the Simply Fit Diet.

Additionally, adopt a weight-reducing eating pattern. Eat breakfast like a king, lunch like a merchant and dinner like a pauper. The best time to be hungry is at night. Strive for variety in the foods you eat. Buy food in season and on sale. Try new foods. To encourage variety, eat at least one vegan meal every six meals.

Quit drinking your calories. If you quit drinking caloric beverages and did not replace those calories with other sources, you could lose 35 pounds a year with no other dietary changes.

The second path of the Simply Fit Diet is to stop eating animal products and wheat. Every other food in the world, including non-wheat whole grains, is available to you on this path. If the universe of food is represented by a watermelon, cut off one end of the watermelon representing junk. Cut off the other end of the watermelon representing animal products, and then make one more slice representing wheat. Toss them. All the remaining food is available to you.

Both paths of the Simply Fit Diet will result in steady, healthful weight loss. But diet alone is not enough. Exercise is an essential component of fitness and you should strive to exercise for an hour a day. If you do not have a favorite form of exercise, try walking, America's most popular activity.

The most common dietary bad habits are alcohol and caffeine consumption. On the Simply Fit Diet you should strive to reduce your bad habits by at least a third, and to confine caffeine to the morning hours and stop drinking alcohol around dinner time.

On the Simply Fit Diet you will obtain abundant nutrition from a wide variety of healthful, natural foods. Absent a special medical need, vitamin and mineral supplements are unnecessary. Also, you should strive to avoid over the counter drugs and other chemicals. When in doubt, take the natural route.

The best diet is one that works, and either path of the Simply Fit Diet will work. The most healthful diet, however, is not as clear. My best guess is that merging the paths of the Simply Fit Diet so that you eat animal products only about once every three to six meals, and that you incorporate whole grains into your diet as tolerated, is the most healthful diet.

If you follow the Simply Fit Diet, you will reach your weight goal. However, once you reach your weight goal, you face a dangerous time. Most dieters regain the weight they lost. By continuing to carefully monitor your weight and by slowly reintroducing eliminated foods into your diet, you can maintain a healthy weight.

Conclusion

I am the fattest kid from a fat family. Fat was my destiny, along with diabetes, cardiovascular disease and other problems. But if you met me today, you would assume that I am one of the lucky, naturally slim people.

While scientists argue back and forth about why we are fat, debating the fat hypothesis and the carbohydrate hypothesis, both as individuals and as a nation we have grown fatter, so now almost 70% of American adults are fat. The science, for all we have come to worship it, is not working. The war on weight began decades ago and no scientific solution has been discovered. It is time for a little common sense. The best diet is one that works. The Simply Fit Diet works.

Good habits like saving and investing money or eating well and exercising take years to pay off. Sometimes, in youth, it seems like the ones who live on charge cards and party all night long are making the right choices. But as the years go by, the wisdom of thoughtful living begins to pay dividends. Past 50, the party people are still living on charge cards and showing physical signs of wear and tear–diabetes, for example; while the careful ones begin to reap the rewards of retirement and the health to enjoy it.

As I put the finishing touches on this book, I have learned that my brother who lost his leg to diabetes has died. He was 64. Although older brothers don't listen much to younger brothers, I secretly hoped this book would help him. Now it is too late. However, his death underscores the importance of making health the most important thing in life. It strengthens my resolve to eat well and exercise.

I would love to tell you that losing weight and becoming fit is easy. I would love to tell you that you can trim down without ever being hungry. I would love to tell you that exercising regularly takes no effort. I would love to tell you there is a magic pill that will make you trim and healthy. But those things are not true. Every day I think about my weight and every day I make an effort to exercise, but the effort is worth it. At age 50, my health was poor, I could hardly run three paces. At age 55, I feel 20 years younger and I am planning a hike to the bottom of the Grand Canyon. The change took work, but the work was worth it.

If being fit is worth a million dollars of health, I have earned $25,000 for each pound I lost. I now possess a million-dollars worth of health. Health is a prerequisite for my goals in life. Health is more important than money. I have been fortunate to be able to improve my health and I want to share what I have learned.

Every day I see people who are so obese, they have trouble walking. I see people whose dietary decisions have lead to diabetes and other diseases. I want to offer them help and advice, but I also want to respect their privacy. Writing this book, The Simply Fit Diet, is my way of resolving this dilemma. The information here is freely available for those who care enough about their health to make an effort to change. I hope this information has helped you and I hope you will share it with others. Thank you.

Visit us online at TheSimplyFitDiet.com

Endnotes

1. The methodology used in establishing the state obesity rates, which are conducted by telephone survey, results in lower reported rates of obesity than actually weighing a sample of the population. The more accurate statistic is that America has an overall obesity rate of 36%. However, the trend toward increased obesity shown by the state maps is instructive.

2. Applebee's Nutritional Information, May 2014. http://www.applebees.com/~/media/docs/Applebees_Nutritional_Inf o.pdf

3. The National Weight Control Registry website, undated. http://www.nwcr.ws/Research/default.htm

4. Metropolitan Life Insurance Company standard height-weight tables for men and women, From the website of Stephen Halls, MD, May 26, 2008. http://www.halls.md/ideal-weight/met.htm

5. Buxton, Orfeu, *et. al.*, "Metabolic Consequences in Humans of Prolonged Sleep Restriction Combined with Circadian Disruption," *Science Translational Medicine*, 4(129), April 11, 2012, reprinted at the National Institutes of Health website, 2012. http://www.ncbi.nlm.nih.gov/pmc/articles/PMC3678519/

6. McDonald's "My Meal Builder" website, 2014. http://www.mcdonalds.com/us/en/meal_builder.html

7. Report of the DGAC on the Dietary Guidelines for Americans, Part D, Section 2: Nutrient Adequacy, 2010. http://www.cnpp.usda.gov/Publications/DietaryGuidelines/2010/DG AC/Report/D-2-NutrientAdequacy.pdf

8. Harvard School of Public Health, "The Problem with Potatoes," *The Nutrition Source*, January 24, 2014. http://www.hsph.harvard.edu/nutritionsource/2014/01/24/the-proble m-with-potatoes/#more-8983

9. Kienzle, Ellen, Bergler, Reinhold, and Mandernach, Anja, "A Comparison of the Feeding Behavior and the Human-Animal Relationship in Owners of Normal and Obese Dogs," *The Journal of Nutrition*, vol. 128, no. 12, 2779S-2782S, December 1, 1998. http://nutrition.highwire.org/content/128/12/2779S.short#T6

10. Jakubowicz, Daniela, Barnea, Maayan, Wainstein, Julio and Froy, Oren, "High Caloric Intake at Breakfast vs. Dinner Differentially Influences Weight Loss of Overweight and Obese Women," *Obesity*, Volume 21, Issue 12, pages 2504–2512, December 2013. http://onlinelibrary.wiley.com/doi/10.1002/oby.20460/abstract

11. Bao Ying *et. al.*, "Association of Nut Consumption with Total and Cause-Specific Mortality," *New England Journal of Medicine*, 369:2001-2011, November 21, 2013. http://www.nejm.org/doi/full/10.1056/NEJMoa1307352

12. Panahi S, El Khoury D, Luhovyy BL, Goff HD, Anderson GH, "Caloric Beverages Consumed Freely at Meal-Time Add Calories to an Ad Libitum Meal," *Appetite*, 65:75-82, June 2013. http://www.ncbi.nlm.nih.gov/pubmed/23402713

13. National Institutes of Health Research Matters, "Risk in Red Meat?" March 26, 2012. http://www.nih.gov/researchmatters/march2012/03262012meat.htm

14. The National Weight Control Registry website, "NWCR Facts," undated. http://www.nwcr.ws/Research/default.htm

15. ESC Press Office, "Ability to Sit and Rise from the Floor Is Closely Correlated with All-Cause Mortality Risk. Test of Musculo-skeletal Fitness Is 'Strong Predictor' of Mortality in the Middle-aged and Older," *European Society of Cardiology*, December 13, 2012. http://www.escardio.org/about/press/press-releases/pr-12/Pages/ability-to-rise-correlated-mortality.aspx?hit=dontmiss

16. Hanson, David, "Alcohol, Problems and Solutions," State University of New York, 1997-2013.
http://www2.potsdam.edu/alcohol/AlcoholAndHealth.html#.U0CYsfldXZg

17. "International Drinking Guidelines," International Center for Alcohol Policies, February 2010.
http://www.icap.org/table/Internationaldrinkingguidelines

18. Peters, Ruth, Peters, Jean, Warner, James, Beckett, Nigel, and Bulpitt, Christopher, "Alcohol, Dementia and Cognitive Decline in the Elderly: a Systematic Review," *Age and Ageing*, Volume 37, Issue 5, Pp. 505-512, 2008.
http://ageing.oxfordjournals.org/content/37/5/505.long

19. Hanson, David, "Alcohol, Problems and Solutions," State University of New York, 1997-2013.
http://www2.potsdam.edu/alcohol/AlcoholAndHealth.html#.U0CYsfldXZg

20. Van Dam, Rob and Feskens, Edith, "Coffee Consumption and Risk of Type 2 Diabetes Mellitus," *The Lancet*, Volume 360, Issue 9344, Pages 1477-1478, November 9, 2002.
http://www.thelancet.com/journals/lancet/article/PIIS0140-6736(02)11436-X/fulltext

21. Huxley, Rachel, *et. al.*, "Coffee, Decaffeinated Coffee, and Tea Consumption in Relation to Incident Type 2 Diabetes Mellitus. A Systematic Review With Meta-analysis." *Archives of Internal Medicine,* 169(22):2053-2063, 2009.
http://archinte.jamanetwork.com/article.aspx?articleid=773949

22. Vinson, Joe, Burnham, Bryan, and Nagandran, Mysore, "Randomized, Double-blind, Placebo-controlled, Linear Dose, Crossover Study to Evaluate the Efficacy and Safety of a Green Coffee Bean Extract in Overweight Subjects," *Diabetes, Metabolic Syndrome and Obesity: Targets and Therapy,* 5:21-27, 2012.
http://www.ncbi.nlm.nih.gov/pmc/articles/PMC3267522/

23. Guallar, Eliseo, *et al.*, "Enough Is Enough: Stop Wasting Money on Vitamin and Mineral Supplements," *Annals of Internal Medicine*, 159(12):850-851, December 17, 2013.
http://annals.org/article.aspx?articleid=1789253

24. Kapis, Vikal, *et. al.*, "Physiological Role for Nitrate-reducing Oral Bacteria in Blood Pressure Control," *Free Radical Biology and Medicine*, 55:93–100, February 2013.
http://www.sciencedirect.com/science/article/pii/S0891584912018229